Classic Yoga *for* Stress Relief

Vimla Lalvani

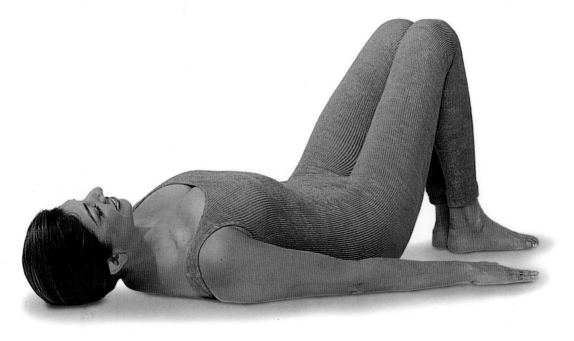

Classic Yoga *for* Stress Relief

Vimla L

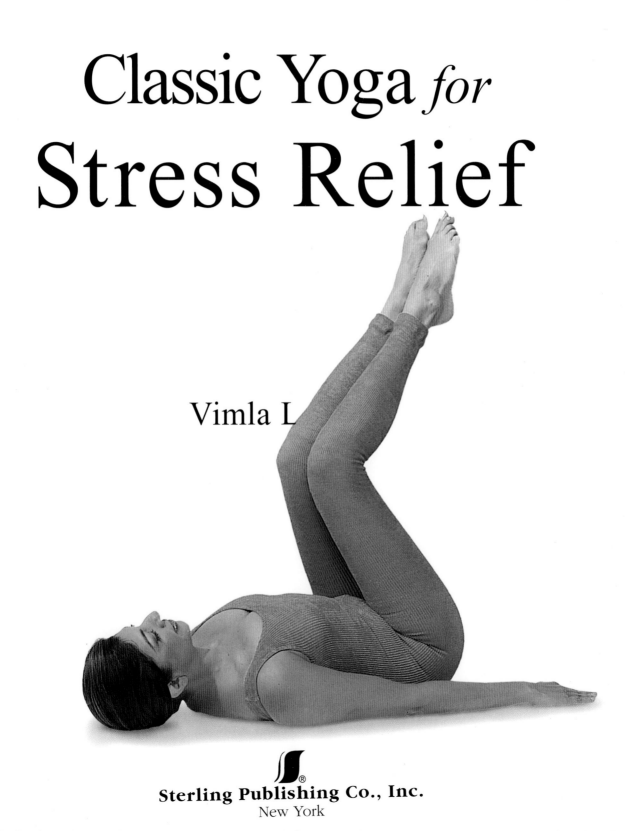

Sterling Publishing Co., Inc.
New York

Contents

SAFETY NOTE It is advisable to check with your doctor before embarking on any exercise program. Yoga should not be considered a replacement for professional medical treatment; a physician should be consulted in all matters relating to health and particularly in respect of pregnancy and any symptoms which may require diagnosis or medical attention. While the advice and information in this book are believed to be accurate and the step-by-step instructions have been devised to avoid strain, neither the author nor the publisher can accept any legal responsibility for any injury sustained while following the exercises.

Remedial Yoga

Library of Congress
Cataloging-in-Publication Data Available

10 9 8 7 6 5 4 3 2 1

Published in 1999 by Sterling Publishing Company, Inc
387 Park Avenue South, New York, N.Y. 10016

Text © The Natural Therapy Company Limited 1997
Design © Octopus Publishing Group Limited 1997
Photographs © Octopus Publishihg Group Limited 1997

Distributed in Canada by Sterling Publishing
c/o Canadian Manda Group, One Atlantic Avenue, Suite 105
Toronto, Ontario, Canada M6K 3E7

The moral right of the author has been asserted.

Printed and bound in China

Sterling ISBN 0-8069-1961-2

Introduction

Yoga and modern living

It's no secret that the pressures of modern living cause stress – and as stress levels continue to rise inexorably the medical profession attempts to reduce them through prescribing sleeping pills and other drugs aimed at promoting relaxation. Yet yoga, which is available to everyone, provides a natural solution, and a longterm approach to dealing with life's many challenges.

When the body and mind are unbalanced the immune system breaks down, allowing illnesses to take hold. Yoga creates perfect harmony by integrating mind, body and soul. While it is generally practiced as a preventive measure, it can also assist in alleviating or curing certain stress-related problems – so even though we cannot avoid today's stress factors, yoga can teach us to cope with them and so enhance the pleasure we take in our daily lives.

What is stress?

Stress is not always a bad thing, as a certain amount gives us challenge and excitement. However, there is a point at which it becomes unhealthy and even dangerous, and it is not always easy for the sufferer to tell when that point has been reached. The body will respond to stress by working harder to cope, until eventually it succumbs to total fatigue, often quite unexpectedly.

When stress overloads the system the levels of the hormones adrenaline, noradrenaline and corticosteroids begin to to rise, and in the short term this gives rise to tense muscles, nausea and rapid breathing and heart rates. If this is ignored, longterm stress sets in – and among the many problems it can cause are allergies, irritable bowel syndrome, panic attacks, depression, insomnia, migraine, asthma, ulcers, colitis, hormone imbalance, high blood pressure and heart disease. A number of other illnesses may be aggravated by it. So while the word 'stressed' is often bandied about, it is in fact not a condition to be taken lightly. Indeed, doctors describe stress as a killer.

Stress may have many causes, and what makes one person feel uncomfortably stressed may make another just feel pleasantly stimulated. However, there are certain major factors that will cause stress to everyone: top of the list is bereavement, followed by divorce, moving house and other lifestyle changes such as a new job. These events have always been with us, but today we also have to cope with an unstable employment market, the scattering of the family structure and mundane but very stressful factors such as increasingly noisy roads, traffic jams and rush-hour commuting on packed trains. It's no wonder we suffer from stress — and no wonder that we search for the peace and relaxation that can be found in yoga.

How yoga works

Yoga is an ancient system of movement developed over 2,000 years ago. The emphasis is to unify the entire system through breathing techniques, gentle exercise and mind control. This combination of practices produces an inner calm and tranquillity that goes deep into the mind and body. The result is a feeling of peace and harmony that translates in the way you think and react to certain situations. When you are relaxed and in control of your thoughts and emotions you are better able to cope with even the hardest problems. Most people panic when faced with difficulties and this increases the stress levels immediately. Just learning to breathe from the diaphragm acts as natural tranquillizer that calms the nervous system instantly.

The gentle movement and deep stretching of yoga improves the circulation and releases the tension in the muscle groups. Twisting and turning the body releases the toxins that build up during stressful moments and breathing deeply relaxes the nervous system as well as increasing the oxygen levels and blood supply to the internal organs. The cleansing and purifying of the bloodstream rejuvenates each cell in the body, which boosts energy levels.

Another aspect of yoga is the visualization and meditation techniques, which help to train and focus the mind. Meditating connects you to your higher self and makes you aware of inner truth. Everybody begins life with strong intuitive powers but loses touch of this natural gift because of the distractions and obligations of the material world. Meditation helps to restore your confidence in yourself and your higher mind and teaches you to rely on yourself to find the correct solutions to your own problems. Although there are five different schools of yoga, all concentrate on the philosophy of reaching spiritual enlightenment through uniting the mind and body. Meditating is an advanced technique that will help you achieve this goal, and with dedicated practice will set you on a spiritual path of increased wisdom and an understanding of the universe and its laws.

The relevance of yoga today

The popularity of yoga has soared in recent years because people are seeking healthier and more longlasting solutions to the stresses of modern living rather than just turning to medication. Yoga is not mere exercise. Even though *hatha* yoga involves *asanas*, or series of postures that build and tone the muscles, it is a discipline that involves dedication to achieve the benefits – so not only do you achieve a well-toned body but you also gain a strength and clarity of mind. It is a practice that you can continue throughout your life regardless of age, and everyone can benefit from it: students who are working towards vital exams, housewives who must cope with looking after children and home, working mothers who try to maintain a career as well, executives who need to stay on top of stressful jobs, and elderly people having to face ageing and retirement. And yoga is a philosophy of life rather than a religion, so it does not interfere with anyone's religious beliefs.

Yoga philosophy believes that all challenges can be solved by building inner strength and character. Everyone's life is full of ups and downs, and the latter can be hard to overcome. Yoga transforms people's lives by teaching them a new way of thinking and viewing the world, giving them an anchor in an increasingly frenetic age.

Stress management through yoga

The way people act in stressful situations differs widely. Much depends on genetic differences, environmental factors, age, sex, marital status, family circumstances, childhood experiences, diet and occupation. Normally, any type of lifetsyle change will produce stress, and if a person cannot adapt to the changed environment exhaustion sets in and then leads to a development of a stress disorder. Genetic factors dictate whether this disorder will affect a particular organ or show as a susceptibility to a particular condition such as diabetes, peptic ulcers or heart disease.

In the Indian medical philosophy known as Ayurvedic medicine, it is believed that well-being does not consist in the the maintenance of good physical health alone but also includes mental and spiritual health. Yoga therapy's unique contribution is that it directly affects the brain, especially the psychic centre from where all psychosomatic stress disorders are initiated. It is for this reason that remedial yoga helps to manage stress-related ailments.

According to Ayurvedic medicine, people can be divided into three categories according to their energy patterns and physical descriptions. *Vata* people have thin, wiry bodies and tend to be very talkative and restless. They are usually intolerant of cold and affected quickly by fears, likes and dislikes. People with *Pitta* constitutions are intolerant of heat and have excessive hunger and thirst. They are highly intelligent and remain very active throughout their lives. Those with *Kapha* constitutions have a well-toned body and are slow in both action and speech. They have less hunger and thirst and are slow to take up anything new. Even though these are broad categories, most people have a combination of these energies.

When environmental factors remain congenial and harmonious to the individual, good physical, mental and spiritual health is maintained. However, if there occurs some unusual, inadequate or excessive interaction between objects, senses, body and mind, the three 'humors' or energies gradually weaken and diseases begin to afflict the body. The factors can be as diverse as climatic change, misuse of the physical body or sudden psychological disturbances. If these changes are of mild or short duration the body will fight back to regain its natural equilibrium, but if they are dramatic or extend over a longer period the person will find it more difficult to return to normality. Instead of trying to find a specific cause and cure for any ailments, yoga therapy treats the body as a whole by improving health in general.

Yoga living

As societies become more affluent, pressure is put upon individuals to succeed. This is the reason why the incidence of certain disorders in the developed and developing countries is increasing at an alarming rate. However, yoga can play an important role in helping society maintain its harmony and balance; people who practice it regularly are more in tune with themselves and their surroundings and lead much happier lives. By learning to integrate their mind, body and soul they have reached a higher level of consciousness and tend to be more gentle in their approach to life. People who suffer from stress, on the other hand, display it in their posture, breathing patterns and facial expressions.

Yoga is for anyone who wants to prolong a youthful appearance and improve quality of life. It is not about abstinence or saying no to all life's pleasures, but about finding moderation in all that you do. You need not change your dietary habits or behavior patterns as long as they are not excessive. Over indulgence, be it in food, alcohol or smoking, burdens the body with a heavy overload and the system is forced to work twice as hard to cope. Maintaining good health by eating a balanced diet combined with yoga practice is a vital part of yoga living. In our chaotic modern world, this ancient philosophy can restore harmony and balance and bring inner peace back to the soul.

How to use this book

The exercises in the Energy Boosters and Art of Relaxation chapters have been designed to form 20-minute and 30-minute programs respectively. These chapters contain 5-minute exercises to bring immediate relief at home, at work, or while travelling. The Remedial Yoga exercises address the ailments that commonly afflict a stressed body and mind, and can be used to prevent and alleviate them.

Safety guidelines

• These exercises are designed for people in normal health. As with any fitness program, if you feel unfit, are pregnant or are suffering from any injury or medical disorder, you should consult your doctor before embarking on these exercises.

• It is important to follow the given order of the exercises within each section and to read through each exercise before starting.

• Never rush the movements or force or jerk your body. Stop immediately if you feel any sharp pain or strain.

• Let your deep breathing relax your body and allow the stretched muscles and ligaments to carry more energy to the muscle fibers.

• In many positions you will notice that the knee remains straight. Do not hyper-extend or lock the knee but lift the muscle above the kneecap to avoid strain or injury.

• When rolling back up to perfect posture, always release each vertebra slowly, one at a time.

• To avoid injury, always keep the knees in line with the toes.

• Do not perform yoga exercises on a full stomach. Allow an interval of four hours after a heavy meal or one hour after a light snack.

• Wear loose, comfortable clothing.

• Exercise in a warm, well-ventilated place.

• All yoga exercises are done in bare feet so that you can grip the floor with your toes. Make sure you practice on an even, non-slip surface. You may find it more comfortable to use a mat for the floor exercises.

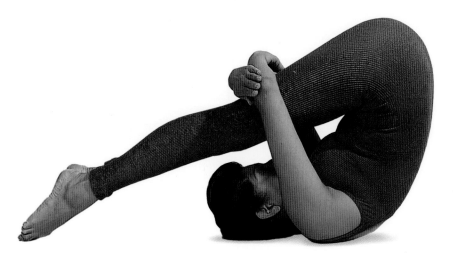

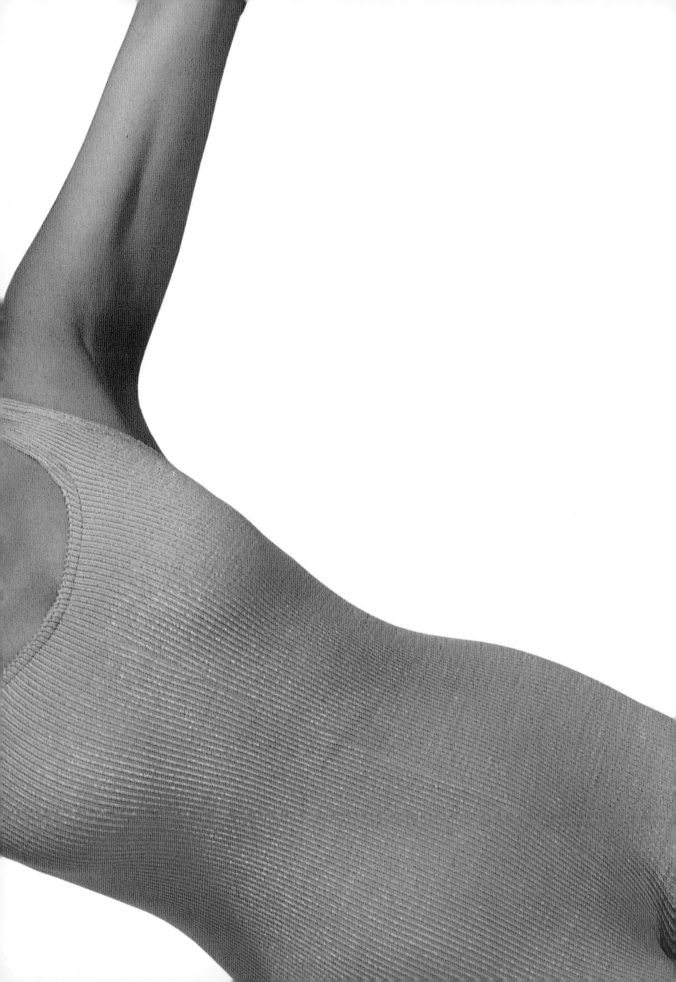

Energy Boosters

People who suffer from stress complain of fatigue, depression and generally feeling unwell. They usually lead sedentary lives with little exercise and seem to have no joy in anything they do; lack of energy affects their mental health and erodes their self-esteem. Acidic diets and diets containing stimulants and medications also deplete the body of energy. Yoga exercise is the best way to boost the body by releasing tension in the muscles as well as improving blood circulation and lymphatic drainage. Deep breathing, combined with stretching, increases the oxygen in the system and rejuvenates all body cells, giving you more energy. When stress is deeply rooted in the muscle groups, any jarring movements can cause injury. Yoga, with its gentle approach, will slowly ease the stress in the body while increasing stamina and strength. Stress can also cause stiffness in the ligaments and joints, and bending forward, backward and sideways can increase your body's flexibility and energy flow. Twisting movements release toxins from the organs, and inverted positions soothe the nervous system. Yoga exercises also lubricate the joints and arteries and build muscle tone as you age. In this chapter I have developed a gentle, easy, safe 20-minute exercise program for people of all ages to release tension, increase energy levels and tone the body. There are also 5-minute energy boosters for home, work and travel to lift your spirits and rejuvenate you.

Breathe and Stretch

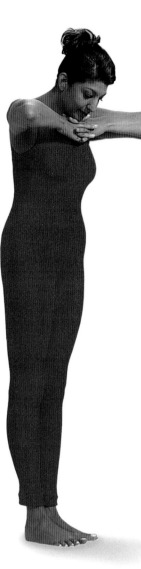

Deep breathing combined with stretching exercises increases your energy flow. As you stretch upward the heart muscle is stimulated, increasing your pulse rate, and the deep breathing improves your blood circulation. This exercise gives you extra vitality and a positive mental attitude, and emphasizes the importance of correct posture. When your feet are placed on the floor, grounding your energy, you can feel it flow through every muscle and nerve as you stretch up. Feel how it flows from the back of your heels up through your knees and thighs to your tailbone. As you move your arms in a circular pattern, feel the energy move up your spine and neck and up through the top of your head into the fingertips.

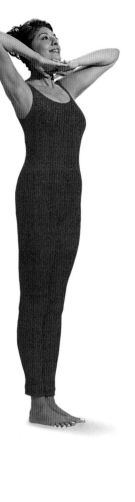

Stand in perfect posture, spine straight and feet together. Keep your shoulders down and chest open with your tailbone tucked in. ▶ Interlace your fingers and put your hands under your chin. Lift your elbows high and look up. ▶ Inhale deeply, drop your chin to your chest and slowly straighten your elbows. ▶ Continue inhaling and bring your arms out in front. ▶ Stretch your arms up, looking toward your hands. ▶ Try to take your arms behind your ears, elbows straight. Exhale and breathe in and out deeply while holding the position. Lift thigh muscles and tighten tummy and buttock muscles. Keep stretching upward; hold for 10 seconds and repeat the exercise.

For perfect posture see page 32.

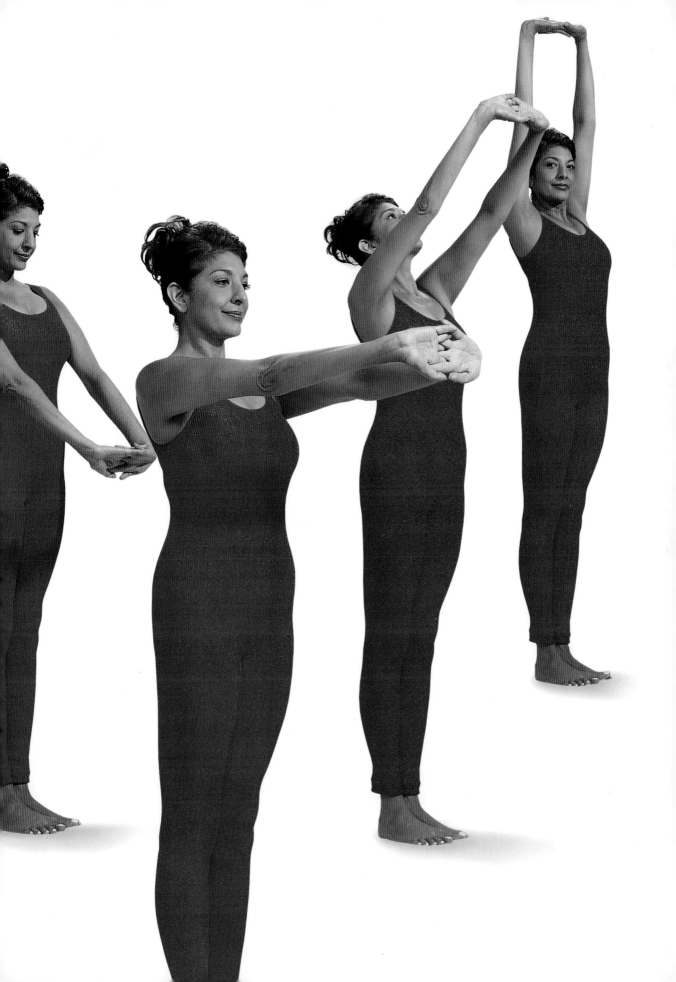

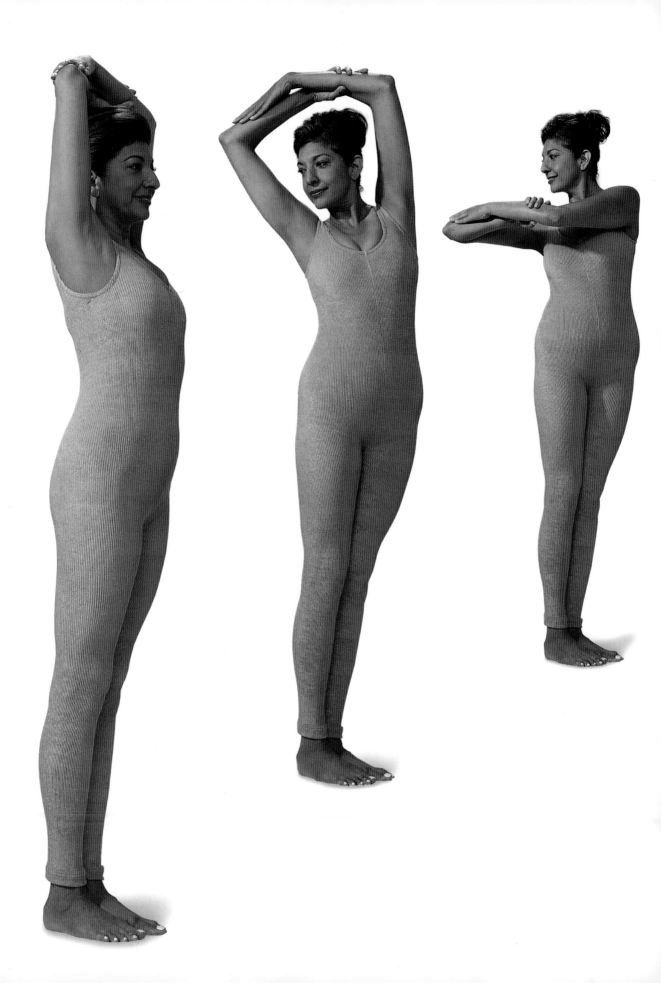

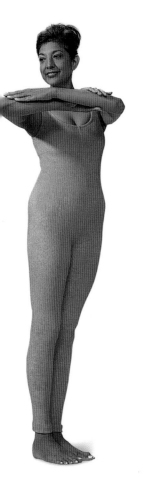

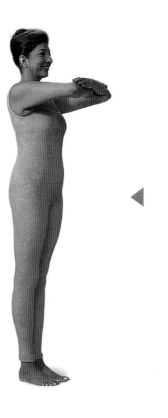

Side Twist

Twists help to improve the flexibility of your spine and release any toxin build-up that has occurred in the body's internal organs. Tension in the back, caused by stress, is released instantly as you slowly twist from side to side. The most important thing to remember while you are doing this exercise is to keep your toes pointing forward and your lower body facing in the same direction, as it is only the upper torso that twists around. By only moving the upper body you increase the depth of the twist and allow the spine to rotate to release stiffness in the back, neck and shoulders. In the beginning you might find that your hips sway sideward, but resist this rotation. As your spine becomes more supple and flexible you will find that you can twist even further around.

For perfect posture see page 32.

Standing with perfect posture, place your left arm on top of your right arm at shoulder height, keeping your shoulders down. ▸ Inhale and slowly turn to the right, keeping your hips and toes facing forward. ▸ Look over your right shoulder; exhale and begin to breathe in and out again even more deeply, turning even further to the right while still looking over your shoulder. ▸ From this position take your arms over your head, still breathing in and out deeply, and hold for a few seconds. ▸ Rotate back to the front, returning to perfect posture but still keeping your arms above your head. Bring arms down and return to start position. Change the arms so that the right arm is above the left and do this sequence again on the left side, twisting over the left shoulder. Repeat the exercise on both sides.

Back Bend

In yoga you bend your body in every direction to free it from any mental or physical blockages. Fear often manifests itself in the body in some form and yoga, with its twisting and turning and forward, sideways and backward movements, can eliminate anxieties and improve total body health. Most people never move backward and are frightened of doing so. Back bends tone up the spine, releasing vital creative energy. They open out the chest, increasing the lung capacity and so enabling you to breathe more deeply. A supple spine gives you a youthful appearance and bending backward increases your flexibility and improves muscle tone. Back bends strengthen the muscles in the lower back and help to alleviate back pain. As you bend, become aware of your body, drawing your energies into yourself.

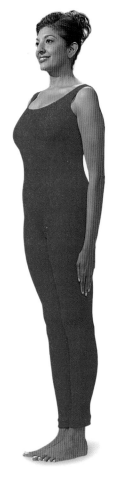
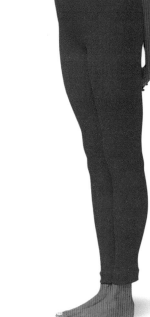

For perfect posture see page 32.

Stand up straight with perfect posture, keeping your arms at your side. ▸ Clasp your hands behind your back, with your shoulders down and elbows straight. ▸ Look upward and slowly push the hips forward as you begin to open the chest. Take your weight onto your heels and clutch the floor with your toes to balance. ▸ Drop your head backward and relax your neck and shoulders. ▸ Breathe deeply and slowly and extend further backward, but do not force your body. Hold for as long as possible, then slowly come back up to the start position. Relax forward to counteract the backbend by bending the knees and dropping your forehead toward them. Move your head to release your neck muscles, and breathe deeply for 5 seconds. Return to standing upright.

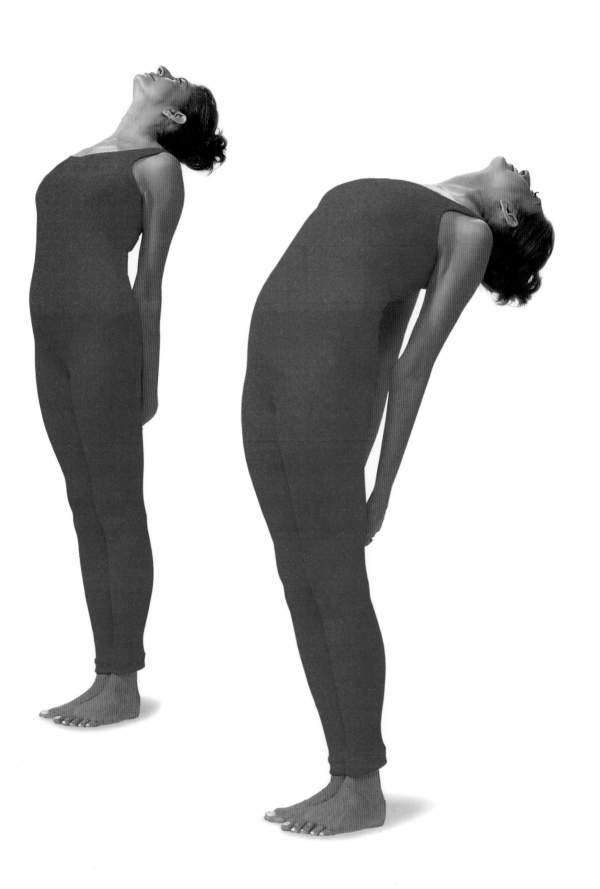

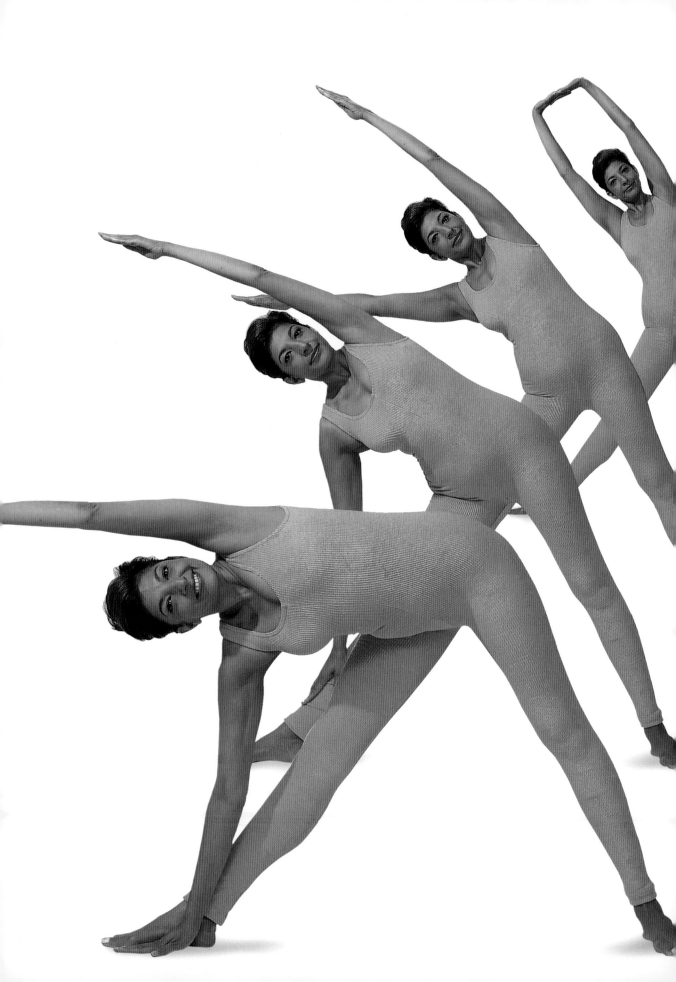

Side Stretch

Stretching to the side helps to strengthen your abdominals and tone up your waist. It improves your body's flexibility and releases any tension in your lower back. Most people never bend or stretch sideways, unless they go to an exercise class, but as the body ages it is very important to stay supple and maintain mobility. As you stretch sideways keep your hips square and facing forward. Try not to twist or turn your hips as you stretch, and keep your feet firmly placed on the floor. Do not collapse your waist but lengthen the spine from the the hip as you extend right down to the floor.

Stand up straight with your feet 1–1.2m (3–4ft) apart, toes pointing forward. Clasp your hands together and stretch your arms above your head as high as possible. Keep your shoulders down and elbows straight. Now turn your right foot to the right. Check your alignment to make sure your right heel is line with the instep of the left foot. Breathe in and out deeply and evenly as you exercise. ▶ Begin to stretch sideways to the right from the waist. ▶ Release your right arm and hold your arms apart for a few seconds. ▶ Place your right hand on your right leg toward your ankle and hold for 10 seconds. ▶ As you improve your flexibility and increase your stretch you will be able to reach all the way down with your palm onto the floor, keeping your arm and hips in a straight line. Release the stretch, stand up straight, and then repeat the exercise on the other side.

Forward Stretch

Stretching forward lengthens the spine and help to calm the nervous system. It opens out the hips and tones up the leg muscles. It is important to lift the muscles above the knees to increase your balance and to enable you to grip the floor with your toes. Always extend your body from the base of your spine while you tighten your abdominal muscles. Some people can feel slightly dizzy because of the increased oxygen in the system, but it passes quickly as you learn to deepen your breathing. As you push your elbows back you will open your chest and release any tension in the neck, shoulders and upper back. In the final position try to concentrate on one point on the floor and keep your back flat in a straight line from the neck to the tailbone.

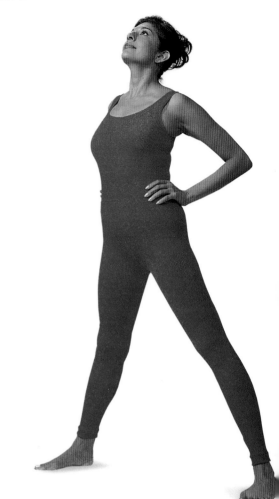

Stand up straight with your feet 1–1.2m (3–4ft) apart and toes pointing forward. ▶ Place your hands on your waist and open out your chest. Inhale deeply and look upward, drawing the elbows toward each other. ▶ Lean forward and point your chin, stretching from the hips and tailbone to straighten the spine. ▶ As you continue to inhale, pause with your back straight and your hips, shoulders and head at a 90° angle. Exhale and hold this position for a few seconds while you breathe normally. ▶ Inhale again and continue stretching downward, exhaling when you have reached as far as you can. Breathe normally and hold this position for 10 seconds. As you deepen your breaths, try to stretch even further without forcing or jerking your body.

When you reach the final position, continue with the exercise on pages 24–25.

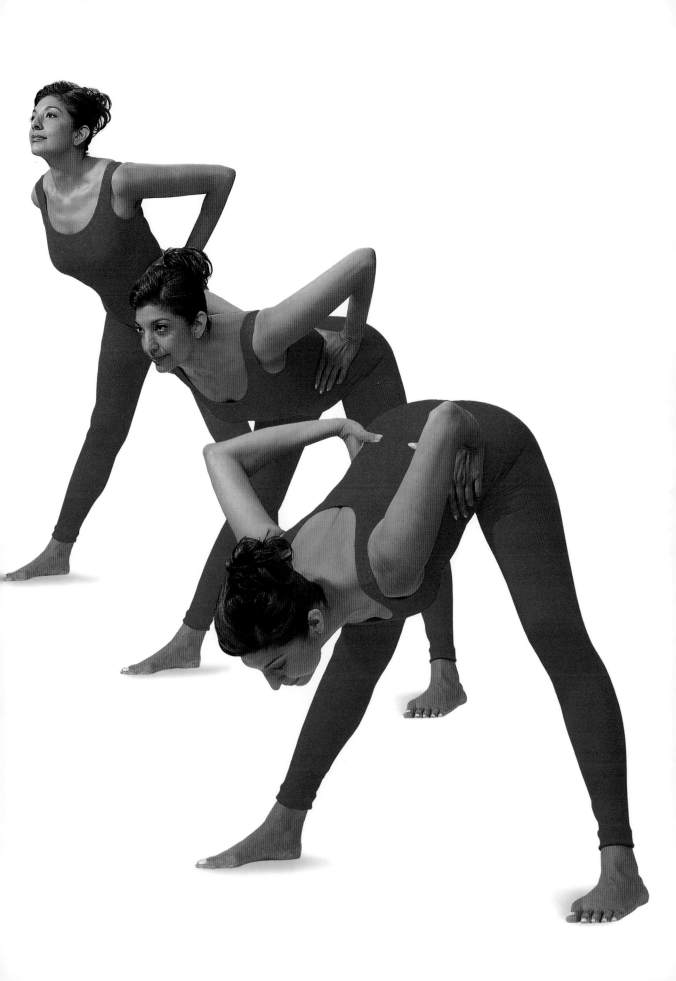

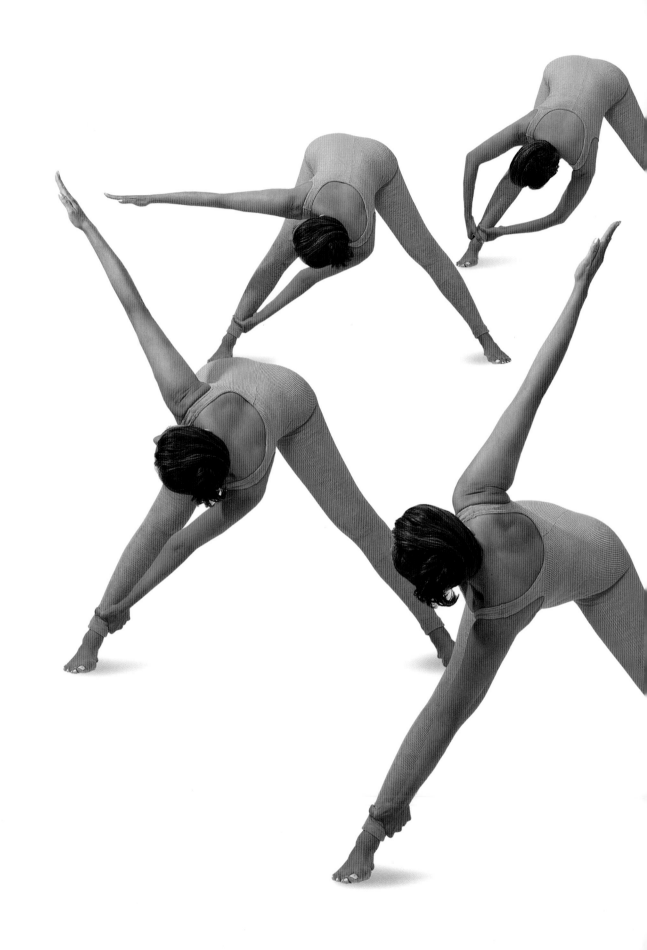

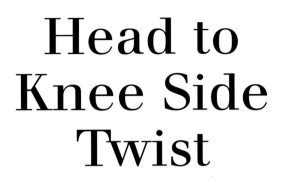

Head to Knee Side Twist

This exercise increases your spine's flexibility, releases toxins from your internal organs and helps back ailments such as sciatica and lumbago. When you take your head forward it helps to soothe your nerves, making you feel calm and relaxed. Suppleness of the spine is essential for good circulation and this exercise combined with deep breathing increases the blood flow through the arteries to boost your energy. When you start to twist, try to turn as far as you can. The final position releases any stiffness you are experiencing in the lower back, neck and shoulders, and also helps to build muscle strength so that you can sit and stand tall.

Continuing from the previous exercise, inhale deeply and as you exhale reach down to your feet, clasping your hands around your ankles. Inhale and exhale deeply for a few seconds to increase the stretch. ▶Now take both of your hands over to the right ankle. If you cannot reach your ankle, take your hands down your right leg as far as you can. ▶ Inhale and take your right arm out to the side in a straight line. Continue to inhale as you start to twist your body around to the back. ▶Look over your right shoulder and continue to twist as far as possible. Exhale and hold this final position for 10 seconds. Return to the start position and repeat the exercise on the other side.

Spinal Stretch

This spinal stretch increases your blood circulation and the flow of oxygen to the brain, helping to relieve tension. It also tones and increases the flexibility of the hamstrings, hips and spine and tones the leg muscles. As you take your arms over your head your breathing pattern becomes shallower, so you have to breathe more deeply to sustain an even pattern. This increase in breathing rejuvenates the body's cells and helps to purify the internal organs. You will experience a tingling sensation in your toes and fingertips as your energy flow is increased. Also your face will glow when you can hold the final position for some time.

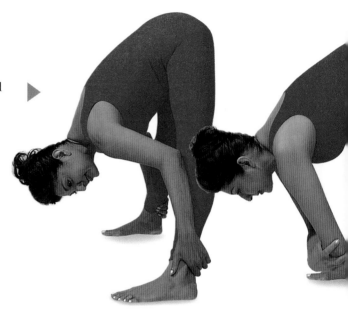

Stand upright with your feet slightly apart, then take hold of your ankles and gently stretch down toward your legs. ▸Cross your arms, holding onto your elbows. Inhale deeply and pull in your abdominal muscles as you begin to stretch your arms over your head. ▸Keep your spine straight and push your hips back behind you. To maintain your balance, shift your weight back onto your heels and grip the floor with your toes. ▸Holding your stomach muscles taut, bring your arms up to your head with your head, neck, shoulders and hips in a straight line. Exhale and breathe deeply, holding this position for 30 seconds. You will feel energized and calmer as you breathe more deeply. To release the stretch, relax your spine and drop your head down toward your feet. Hold for a few seconds.

When you reach the final position, continue with the exercise on pages 28–29.

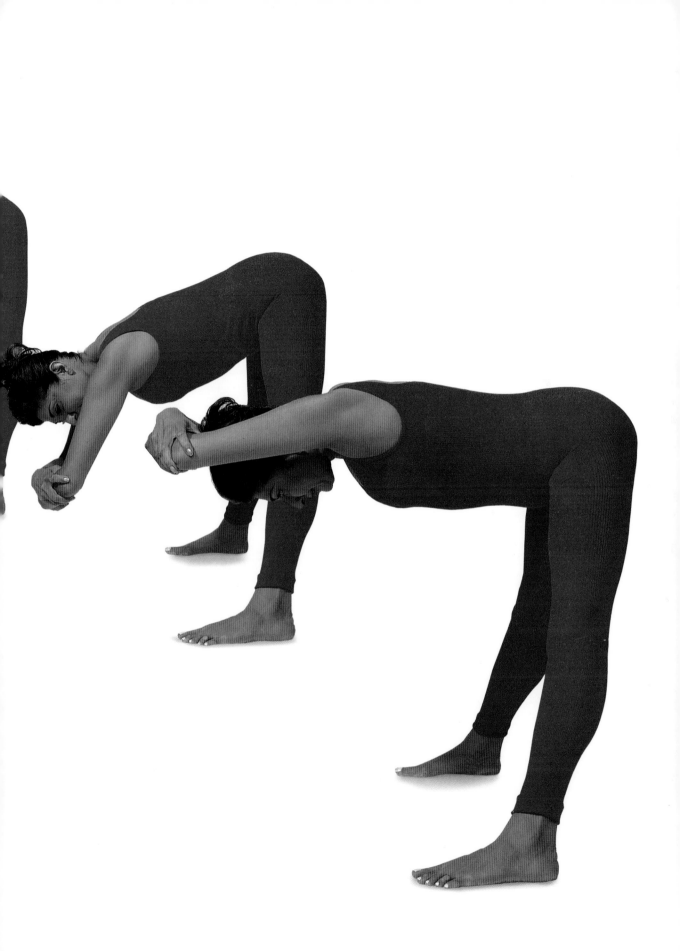

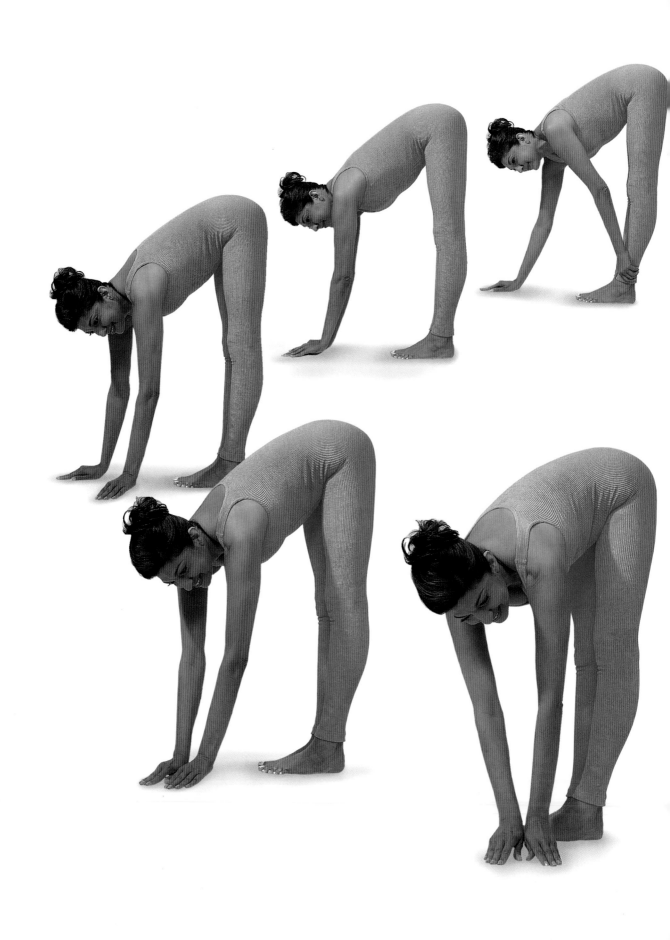

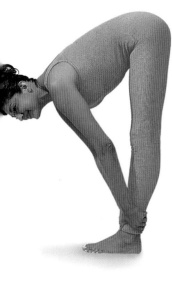

Hip Opener and Twist

It is very important that you increase the flexibility of your hip joints so that your spine mobility improves. People who feel very stressed often complain of feeling lethargic and depleted of energy. This exercise will help open the hips to release muscle tension as well as toxins that are trapped in the kidneys, liver and spleen. Do not allow your hips to move from side to side. It is important to keep the hips square. If you need to bend your knees to reach the floor make sure your feet stay together and your toes point forward. Always be aware of your tummy muscles and hold them up as you stretch forward and twist slowly from side to side.

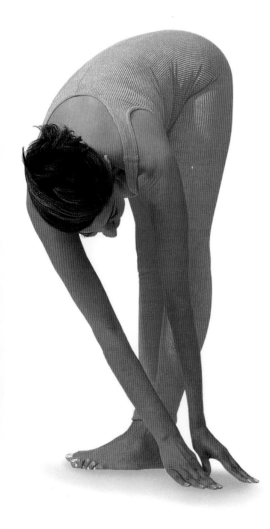

Continuing from the previous exercise bring your feet together and tighten all your leg muscles. Hold your tummy muscles in and grip both ankles with your hands. Breathe deeply and evenly throughout the exercise. ▶Keeping your left hand on your left ankle, place your right palm on the floor in front of you. ▶Then place your left palm on the floor. ▶Slowly begin to twist your hands to the left, taking the left palm first and then the right hand to join the left. Try to keep the elbows straight. ▶Keep twisting to the left and bring the hands close to the feet. ▶To increase the twist take your hands further back toward your heels. Your stomach should rest on your upper thigh as you keep twisting back as far as possible. Return to the start position and repeat the exercise on the other side.

Head to Knee

This bending posture promotes total body health because it allows the energy to flow through the entire system. Not only does the exercise soothe the brain but harmful toxins are also eliminated from the body's organs as the head bends forward. The spine becomes more flexible and supple, which gives you a feeling of elation. This posture also stimulates the sciatic nerve and strengthens the muscles of the lower back. Always gently lengthen the spine forward – never force your body or jerk into the pose. Breathe deeply as you relax forward, eventually trying to stretch out your entire spine as you clasp your ankles.

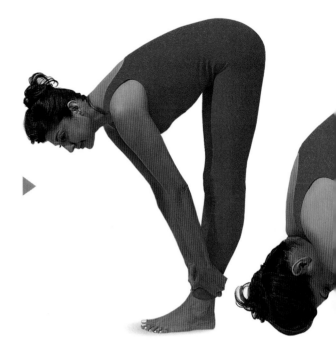

Stand up straight and bring your feet together, then lean down and hold onto your ankles with both hands, keeping your elbows straight. ▸Pulling your tummy muscles in, inhale deeply, bend your elbows and slowly stretch your forehead toward your knees. ▸Exhale and pull your head further down. ▸Breathing deeply and slowly, lengthen your spine as you try to touch your knees with your forehead. Hold the position for 30 seconds. Do not become discouraged if you cannot reach down very far. With continued practice you will be amazed at how far down you can reach.

Think of your spine as circles of energy around the vertebrae and not a solid mass. This will help the way you approach this position as you ease softly and gently down.

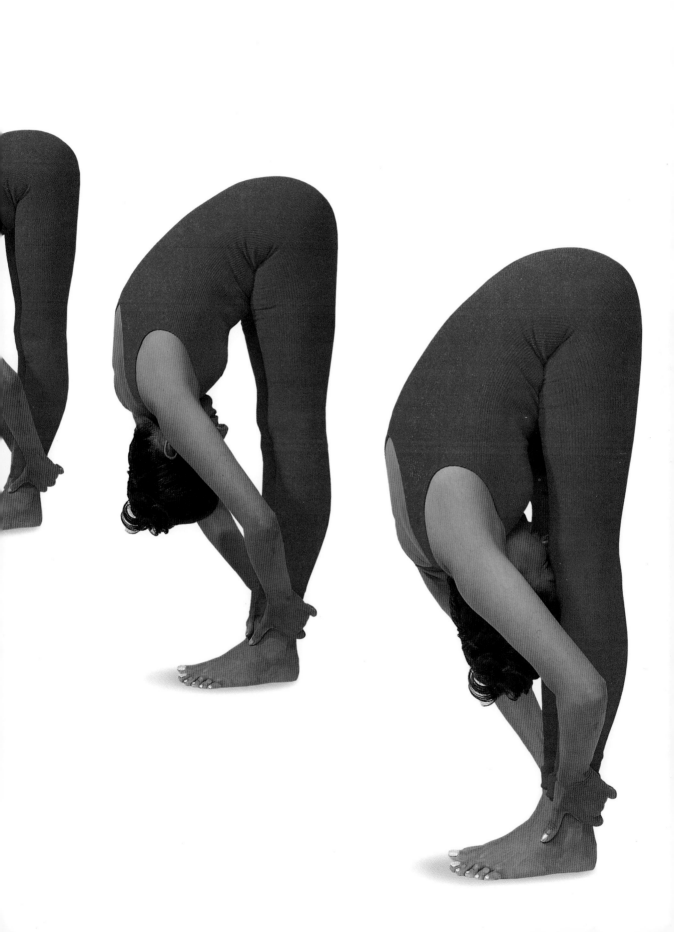

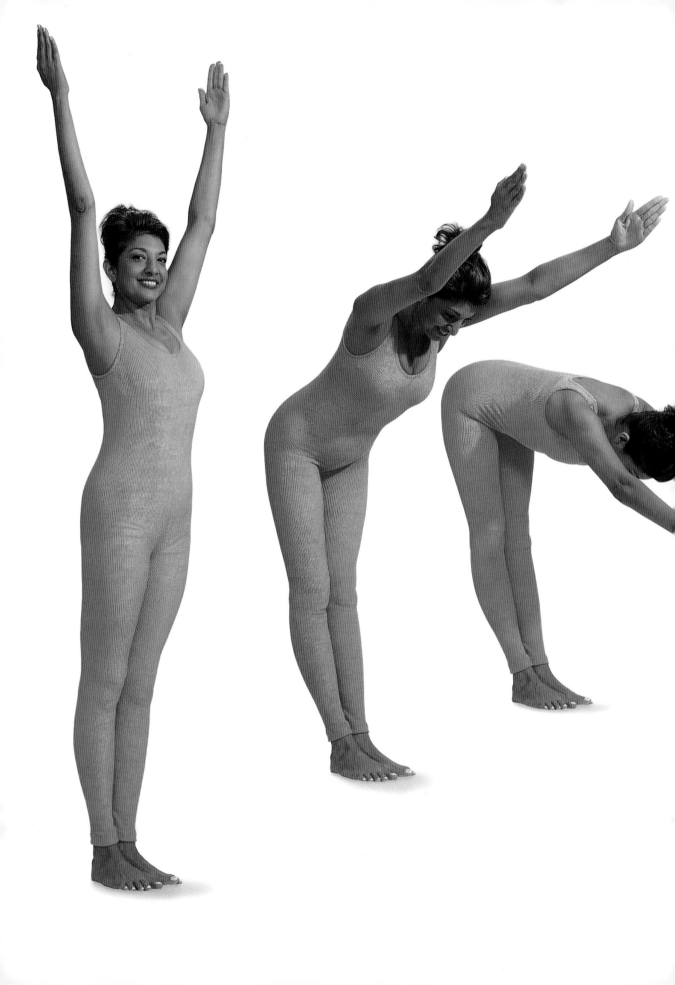

Perfect Posture

It is vital to understand good body alignment and to learn how to sit and stand in perfect posture. Bad posture leads to back ailments, a negative mental outlook and depleted energies. When you are standing and sitting correctly you can breathe properly to your full lung capacity. Most people with bad posture never experience the joy of feeling full of vitality. Stretching in perfect posture aligns and balances the muscles and corrects the tilt of the pelvis. It allows the spine to stay erect so that the body's energy flows freely. By stretching your arms over your head you open out your chest and your hips are free, giving more space for the internal organs to function properly.

Stand upright with feet together and big toes touching and try to balance. Distribute your weight evenly between your heels and toes and grip the floor with your toes. Place your hands on your ankles with your head tucked in. ▶Inhale deeply, straighten your arms and pull up halfway. ▶Then bring your arms out in front of you close to your ears, tightening your tummy and buttock muscles. ▶Keep stretching your arms outward with a straight spine as you stand up. ▶Lift your arms above your head, exhale and breathe normally. Keep your head lifted, your neck extended and your breastbone stretched upward. Then lift your diaphragm, rib cage and abdomen, and tuck in your tailbone; tighten your leg muscles. Release your arms down and stand for 30 seconds, drawing your energies into yourself.

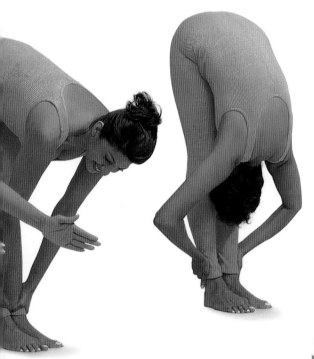

As you stretch up do not hyper-extend your knees by pushing them backward, but lift the muscles above your knees.

Deep Bend

Flexible hip joints help to correct any pelvic imbalance and improve mobility as we get older. This stretch looks simple to do, but it really is a dynamic movement which creates poise and confidence. Keeping your spine upright in perfect alignment while you bend helps you breathe more deeply, but holding the pose can be quite strenous. As you lunge sideways, make sure your knee does not extend right over your foot as this can cause knee strain. The movement should create a 90° angle from the upper body to the back of the knee and heel.

Stand upright with your feet 1.2m (4ft) apart, your toes pointing forward and both hands on your waist. Turn your left foot to the left, keeping the instep of the right foot in line with the left heel. Place your left hand on your left leg with your fingertips on the inner thigh above the knee. Keep your spine straight and hips square, and remember to breathe deeply and evenly throughout the exercise. ▶ Bend your left knee to turn the thigh and hip joints. If the knee moves beyond the foot, take the right leg out further to create a 90° angle. ▶ Now extend the lunge further by pushing the pubic bone down toward the floor, keeping the right leg straight. Push the right foot down toward the floor, tightening the muscle above the knee. Keep your pelvis straight and your breastbone lifted. Enjoy the elation of the stretch, while holding for 10 seconds or more. To release the pose return to the start position and repeat the exercise on the other side.

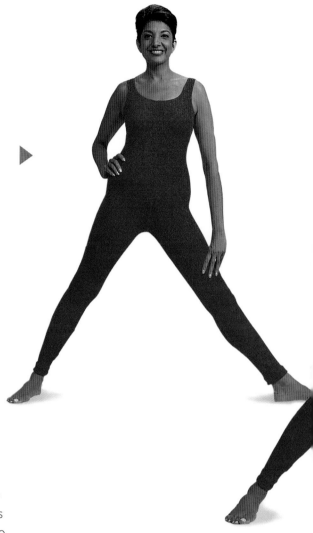

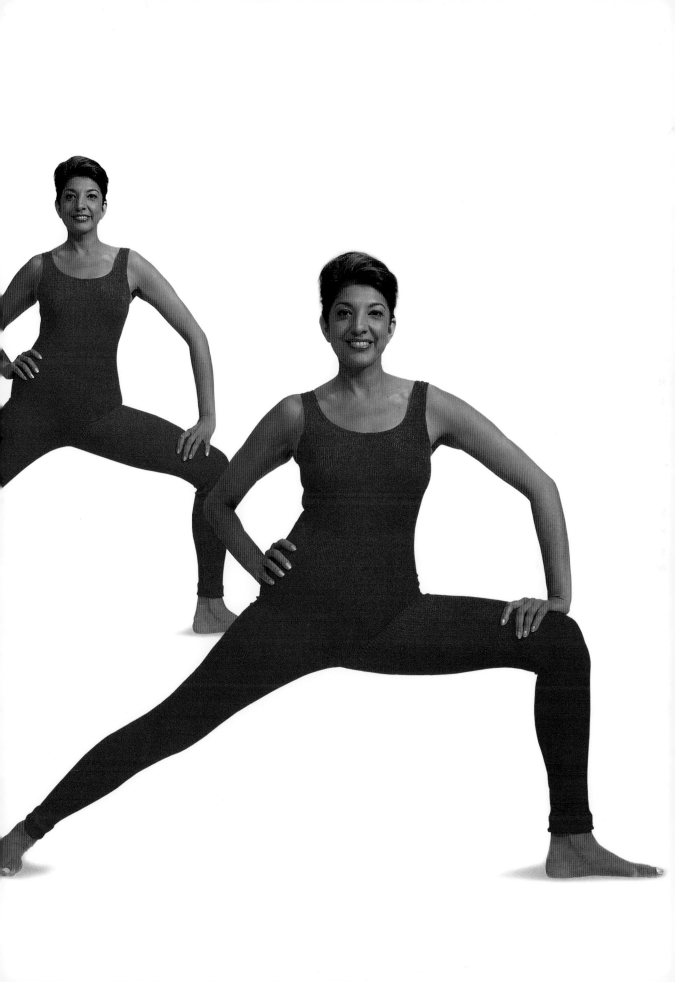

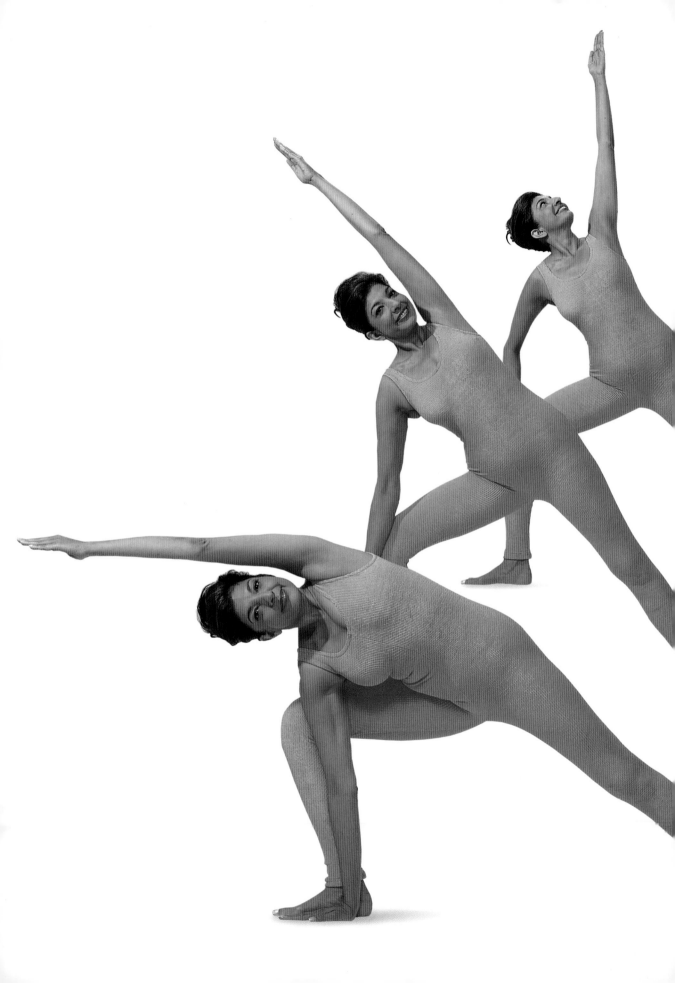

Extended Deep Bend

◀ Extending the arm in this deep bend elongates the waist, increases the body stretch and deepens your breathing. It is important not to collapse your trunk forward but to keep your spine very straight. This helps to strengthen the muscles in your lower back and abdomen and prevent or alleviate back pain. By taking deep and even breaths you send fresh oxygen throughout your system and boost your circulation. This is a wonderful toning exercise for the entire body. As you stretch sideways, remember to stretch from the hips, not from the waist. Feel the stretch from your left foot up through your spine right into your left palm and fingertips.

Begin in the same position as the deep bend (see page 34) but place your right arm on your right leg and extend your left arm out to the side, palm facing upward. ▶Keep the 90° angle between your upper and lower body and inhale deeply, taking your arm up in a straight line. Turn your head up to look at your palm. ▶Exhale and take your arm sideways, turning your face forward and sliding your right hand down your leg. ▶Slide your right hand to the floor in front of your right foot and stretch into the full extension, breathing deeply and evenly. Drop your pubic bone down with your trunk facing forward. Keep your head in line with the spine and your left leg firm. If you start to wobble, tighten the muscles above your left knee and dig your right heel into the floor. Hold still for 20 to 30 seconds and repeat on the other side.

Deep Lunge Balance

This exercise helps to build stamina and muscular strength in your body while teaching you how to clear and concentrate your mind. All balancing exercises take more energy than you imagine and are a great challenge. Most people believe that they are unable to achieve such a difficult final position, but feel a great sense of achievement when they master standing on one leg without shaking. If your mind wanders for even one moment you will start to fall over, so it is important to focus only on achieving your goal. Keep the whole movement fluid because if you pause too long before you start to lift your leg, you may start to lose your balance.

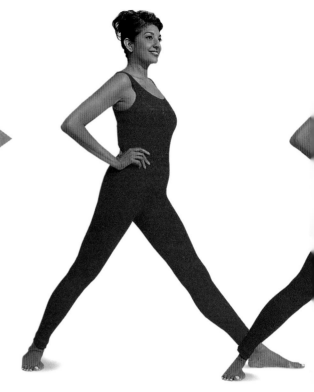

Stand upright with your feet 1–1.2m (3–4ft) apart, facing forward. Turn your right foot to the right so that the instep is in line with the left heel. Turn your upper body so that your hips are square and your breastbone is in line with your knee. ▶Breathing normally, bend your left knee and lunge forward. ▶Straighten both legs, point your right foot behind you, and focus on one spot on the floor to prepare to balance. ▶Inhale deeply and lift your right leg off the floor as you bend forward. Exhale, and breathe normally as you straighten both legs, while keeping your shoulders and hips in a straight line. Hold for as long as possible and bend your left knee to finish. Return to the start position and repeat the exercise on the other side.

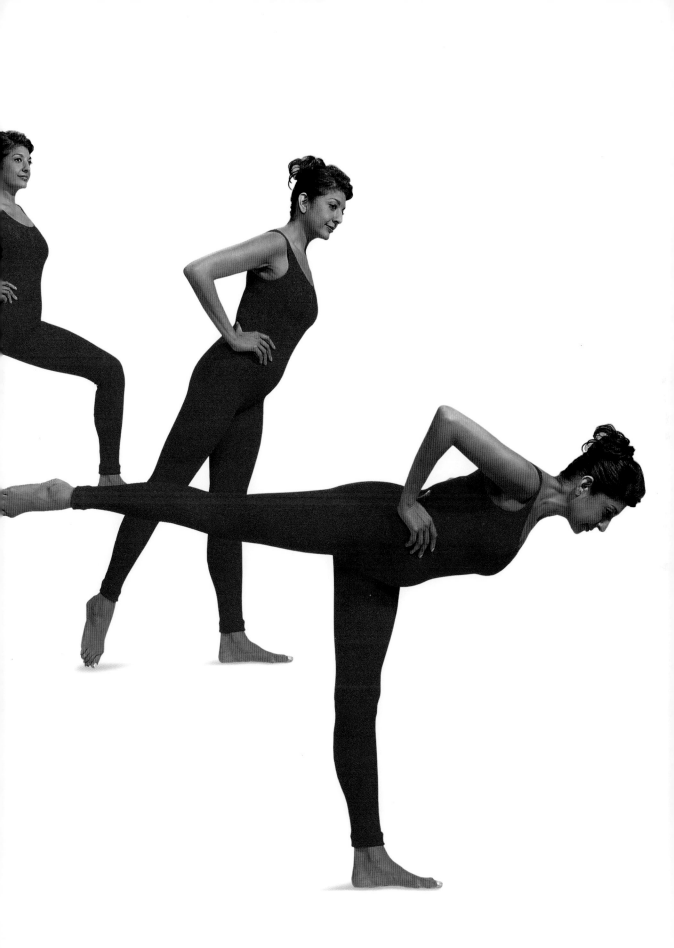

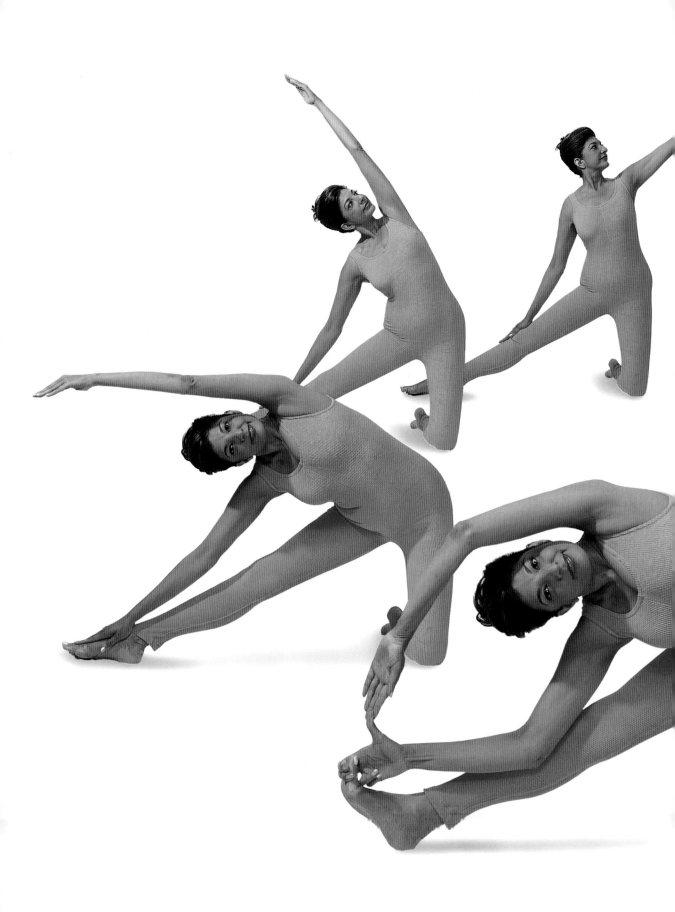

One Knee Side Stretch

Stretching to the side while balancing on one knee increases the flexibility of your spine and also tones the internal organs. There is no opportunity to massage your organs but stretching sideways, combined with some deep breathing, helps to cleanse and purify them, particularly the kidneys, liver and spleen. By increasing the suppleness and flexibility of the spine you can boost your body's energy levels and also stretch the pelvic region. This type of stretch keeps the abdominal muscles and organs in peak condition and releases any stiffness in the lower back.

Kneel on the floor with both knees and ankles together. Stretch your right leg out to the right to line up with the knee of your left leg. Turn the right foot sideways toward the right, keeping the knee straight. ▶Inhale and take your left arm upward and look toward the palm. ▶Lifting your head upward, slowly bend toward the right side. ▶ Sliding your right hand down to your ankle, extend the stretch further. ▶Exhale and continue to breathe normally as you increase the stretch. Bend the first two fingers of your right hand and clasp your big toe while you flex your thumb. Reach your left arm over to touch your thumb with your fingertips. Breathe deeply and evenly and hold for 20 to 30 seconds. Repeat the exercise on the other side.

Camel

This intense back stretch helps to rejuvenate the spine and builds up the muscles in your lower back. It relaxes and soothes the central nervous system while releasing all the muscular tension in the spine which has been caused by stress. It is also a wonderful stretch for your face and neck as the increased circulation to these areas helps to prevent ageing. Many people find it hard to achieve this position and carry some of their body weight in their legs instead of fully extending their hips forward. By doing this the total movement can be restricted. When your body is in perfect alignment it should feel light and compact. Keep extending your hips forward to increase the intensity of the back stretch. Relax your throat and open out your chest, while continuing to breathe deeply throughout.

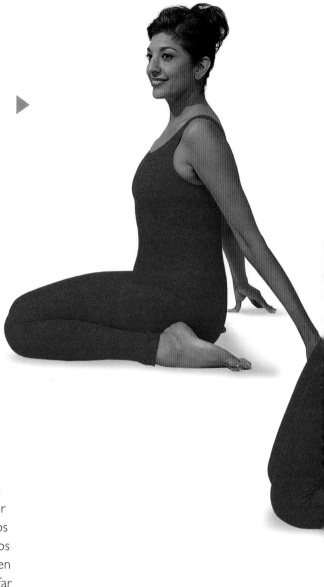

Kneel on the floor, bringing your knees together with your heels close to your hips on either side of your body. Place your fingertips on the floor behind you for support. ▶Inhale and lift your hips and face upward. Now push your knees and hips forward until your weight shifts upward. Open out your chest and throat and relax back as far as possible, still pushing forward with your hips. ▶Create a beautiful circle with your spine and bring your arms in to clasp your heels with your hands. Exhale. Keep extending the hips further to increase the intensity of the stretch. Relax your jaw and the muscles around your eyes. Breathe in and out deeply while you tone your entire spine.

When you are fully extended say 'Aah' to test that all the muscles of your face, especially the jaw, are totally relaxed.

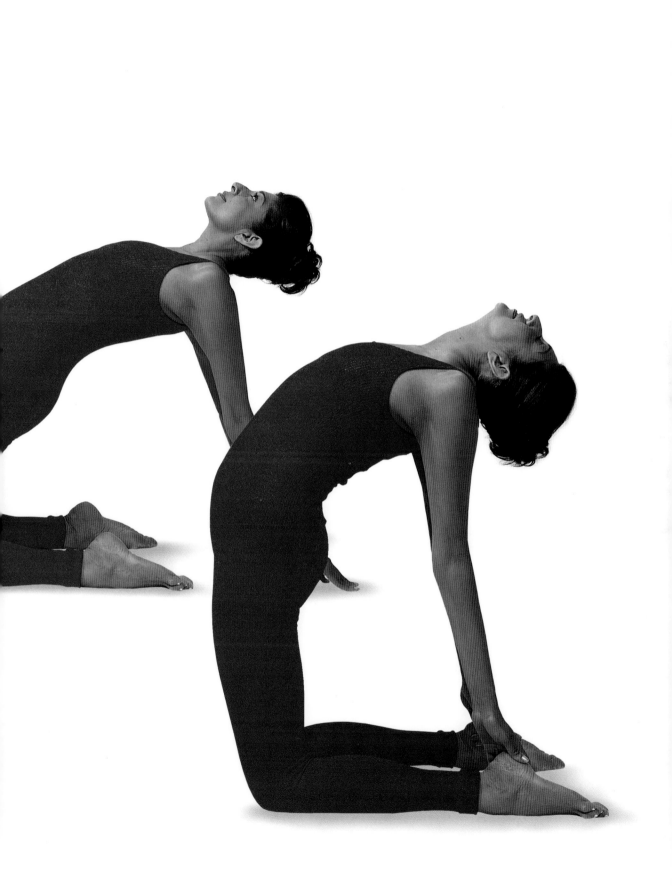

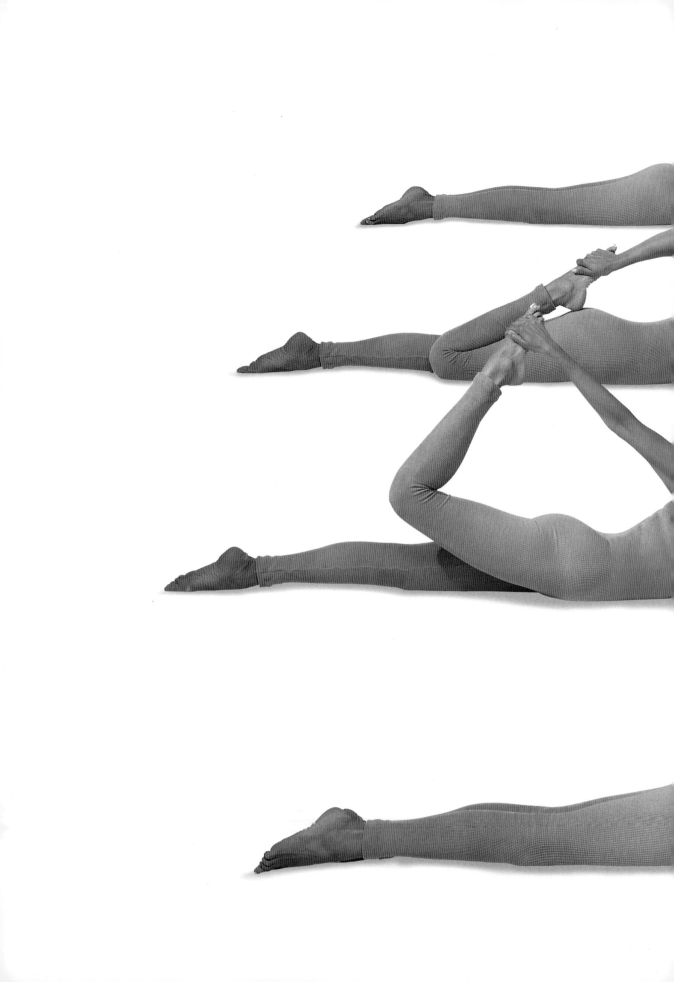

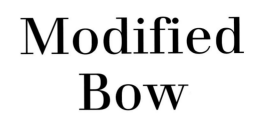

Modified Bow

This exercise releases any tension and stiffness in the lower back and helps strengthen the muscles in this area to alleviate back pain. It tones the leg and buttock muscles and makes you feel very graceful. Because of the position of the abdomen on the floor the internal organs are massaged and invigorated, which in turn helps digestive and bowel disorders, such as a stomach upset and irritable bowel sydrome. The exercise also aids digestion. Taking the head backward is a panacea for displaced spinal discs as it helps to restore them to their original position. The spinal region is toned up, and your chest is expanded to ensure a good energy flow.

Lie on your stomach on the floor with your legs together and arms outstretched in front of you, your palms facing down. Point your toes.

▶Inhale and bend your right leg. Hold on to your toes with your right hand and pull your heel down toward your right buttock. Exhale and hold briefly to feel the stretch in the hamstrings.

▶Inhale and stretch your leg up to create a bow shape. Keep your left leg and hip on the floor. Look upward, but do not strain your neck.

▶Release your leg and return to the start position, then take both arms out in front of you with palms facing and with your elbows turned outward. Inhale, pushing both palms into the floor, and raise your chest, looking upward. Keep your hipbones down and tighten the buttock muscles. Exhale and come back to the start position. Repeat the exercise on the other side.

Cat Stretch

This is a wonderful exercise to relieve all the tension that accumulates in the spine. It also helps to calm the brain and relaxes the neck and shoulders. If you suffer from headaches and backaches caused by stress, you will find that if you place your head down on the floor in this curved position it will help to alleviate the pain. Combined with deep breathing, this exercise soothes your central nervous system and helps you to restore harmony and balance to your life. It slows down your pulse rate and gives you time to escape from any mental anxieties by relaxing the brain so that you find inner calm.

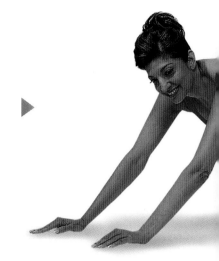

Begin by kneeling down on all fours on the floor and stretch your arms out in front of you. ▶Inhale deeply and begin to drop your hips back toward your heels. ▶Exhale and push your hips all the way down so that your chest rests on your knees, bending your elbows and dropping your head forward to the floor. ▶Breathing in and out deeply, slide your arms back toward your heels. ▶Curl your spine and relax down onto your forehead, sliding your hands back beyond your heels with your palms facing up. Hold until you feel totally relaxed. Do this exercise to rejuvenate yourself if you are feeling tired or lethargic, or use it to shut yourself off from the rest of the world. You can drift into peaceful sleep by turning to one side and rolling over to stretch out your legs.

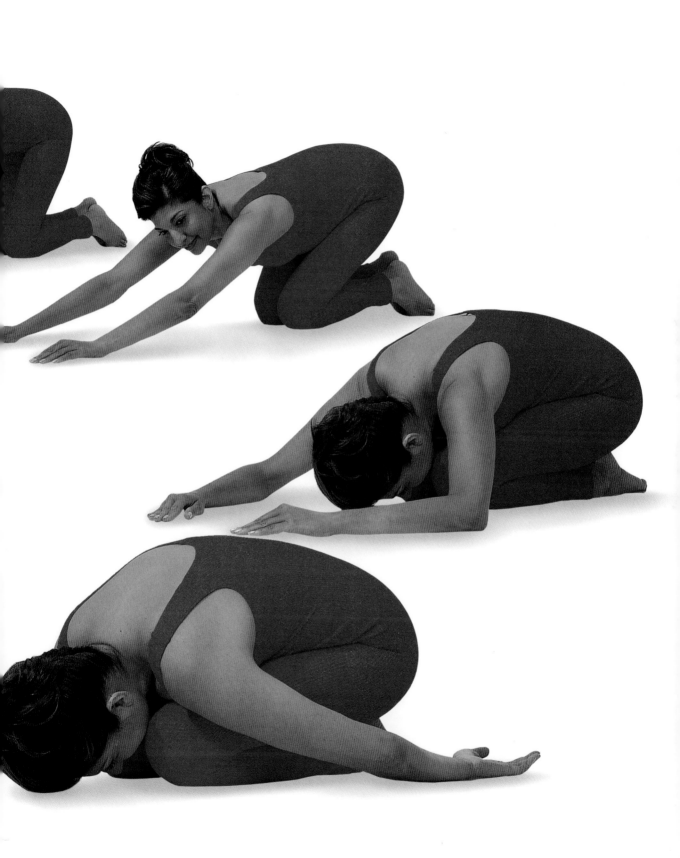

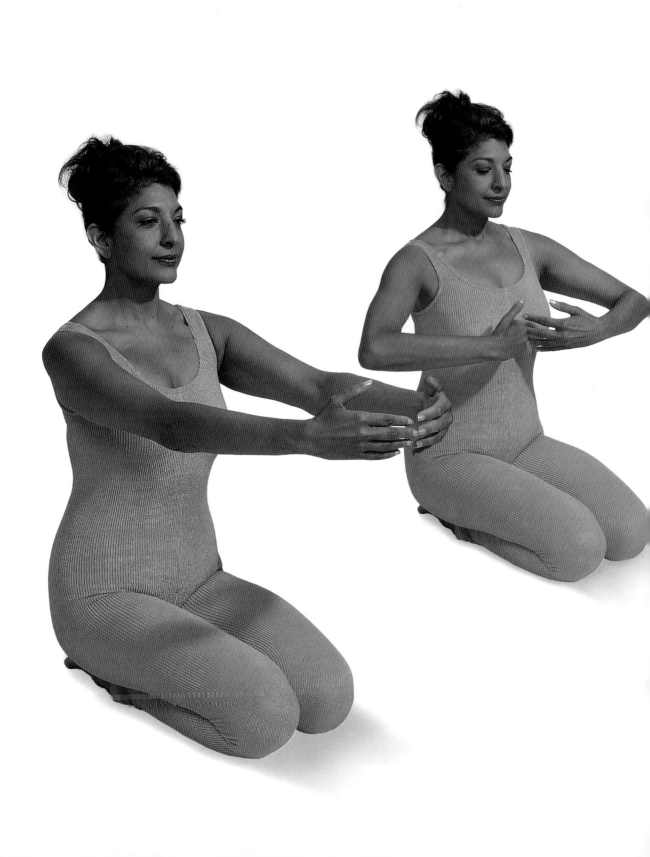

Pranayama

Pranayama is a Sanskrit word meaning 'the science of breath'. It teaches you breath control, which helps to discipline your mind. In yoga we breathe through the nose from the diaphragm. When you are sitting or standing in perfect posture and breathing correctly you will increase your energy levels and revitalize every cell in your body. Breathing from the diaphragm also acts as a natural tranquillizer to calm and soothe the nervous system. When you watch babies and animals breathe you will notice that they breathe naturally from their diaphragms, but at some point as we grow up we forget how to breathe correctly. First of all, pay attention to how you are breathing right now. Most probably you are lifting your chest with your shoulders overextended backward. This allows only a shallow breath which fills just half of your lungs, giving you half the energy. Because of all the fresh oxygen that enters into the system, some people feel dizzy when they first start breathing deeply.

Kneel on the floor, sit up, and straighten your spine. Place your hands on your knees. Just concentrate and observe your present breathing pattern. ▶Take your hands to your diaphragm in front of your belly button, and as you inhale your tummy should move outward. ▶Feel your lungs fill with oxygen and move your arms up to your chest. ▶Then extend them outward in front of you. As you exhale your tummy moves in, so bring your hands slowly back to the first position. Continue to take at least 10 deep breaths until you always breathe from the diaphragm.

HOME:
Body Rolls

When your body stiffens and tenses with stress your spine feels locked. Your normal mobility is blocked and you experience aches and pains throughout your body. The best exercise to relieve this stress is body rolls, as the movements release tension and boost energy levels. Combined with correct breathing the exercise increases your vitality and improves your circulation. While you are breathing deeply and moving your body in a circle the fresh oxygen moving through your body revitalizes, cleanses and purifies the internal organs. Some people feel dizzy in this pose because they have too many toxins in their body. Body rolls are easy to do at home, improve your balance, and encourage a sense of wellbeing.

Stand up straight with your feet pointing forward 1m (3ft) apart. Take your hands to your waist and open out your chest. ▶Inhale and stretch your body to the right, keeping your knees straight. Do not drop your head but keep it in line with your neck. ▶Still inhaling, push your hips forward and extend your head backward, relaxing your neck and shoulders. ▶Exhale and stretch your body to the left. ▶Now flatten your spine and turn your body toward the floor, looking downward. ▶Still exhaling, move forward between your legs and extend down toward the floor. Inhale and return to the start position. Repeat the exercise on the other side. Some people have more tension and stiffness than others, so continue the rolls until you feel your body starting to rejuvenate with energy.

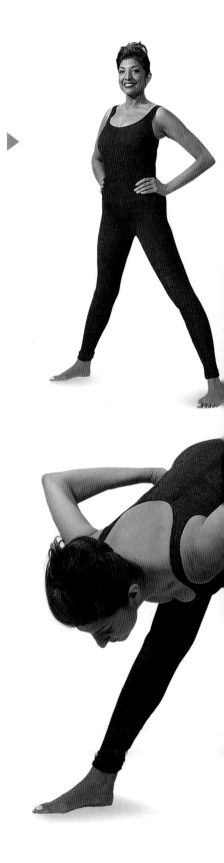

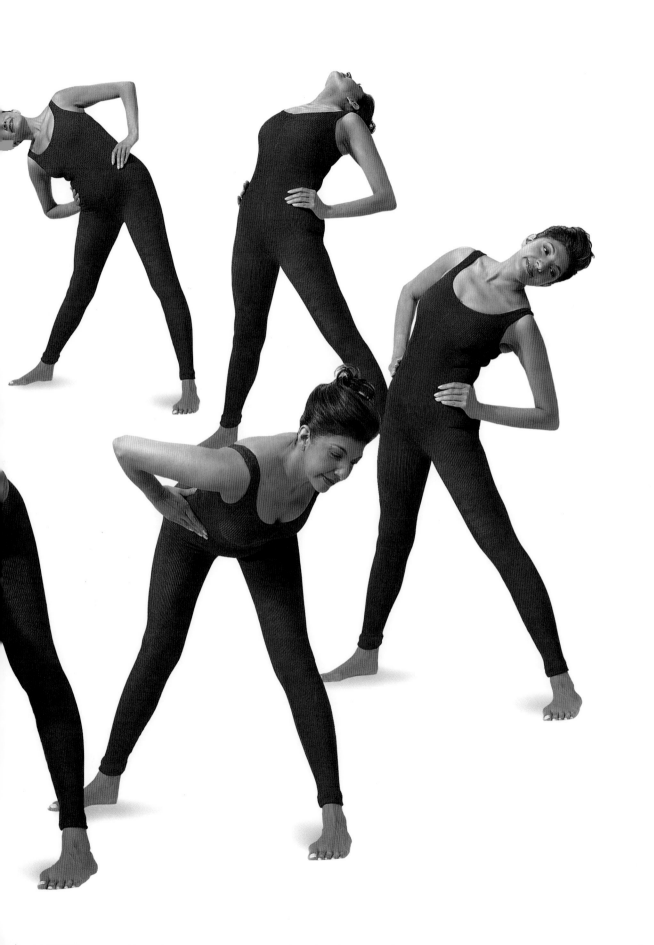

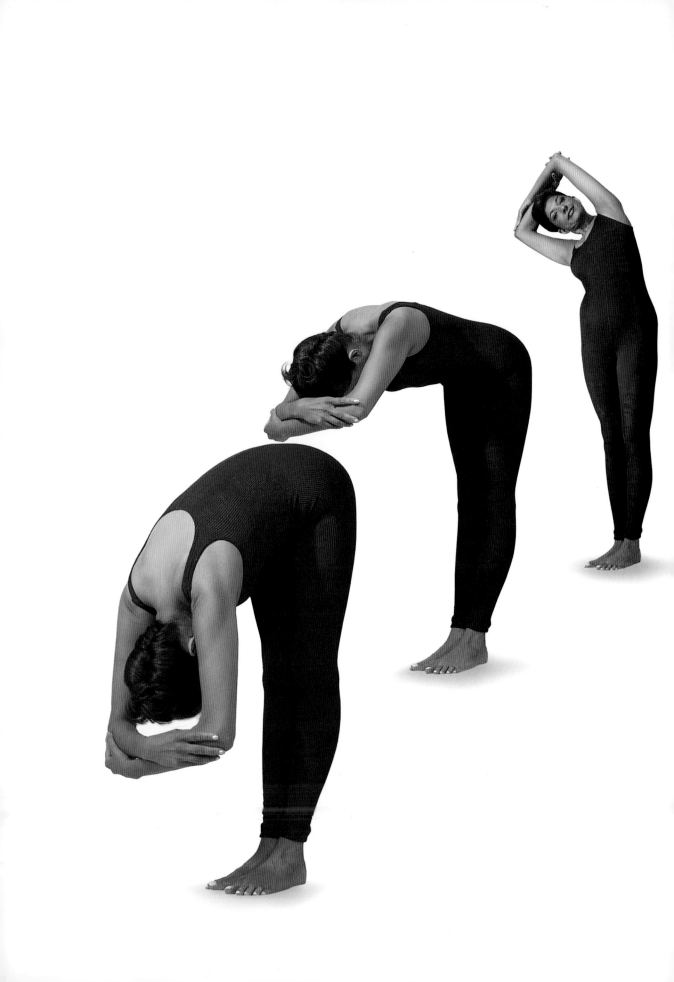

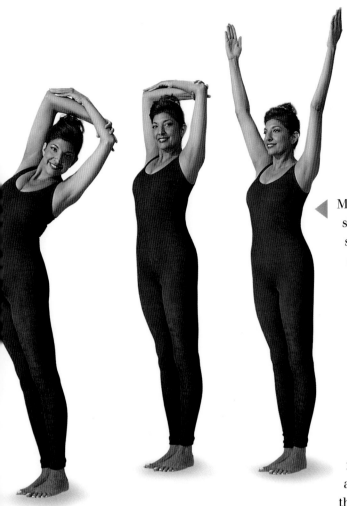

WORK:
Slow Stretching

◄ Most people spend their working day slouched over a desk and consequently suffer from backache, fatigue, boredom and a sense of failure if they cannot cope with their workload. The best way to change these reactions is to boost the energy levels and calm the nervous system. Tension and stress stay in your body until they are consciously removed. If left, your body will seize up and your spine will become immobile. The way to avoid these symptoms is to find a suitable place in your office to do this exercise to release tension and restore mental harmony. Stretching up releases muscular tension in the neck and shoulders and bending forward soothes and revitalizes the nervous system.

Stand up straight with feet together, inhale deeply and throw your arms above your head with palms facing. Keep your shoulders down and your head centered between your arms. Exhale and hold briefly. ►Cross your arms, hold onto your elbows and push your elbows behind your ears. ►Inhale and as you exhale stretch over to the left from the waist with hips and feet forward. Breathe normally and hold briefly. Inhale and return to the center again. ►Exhale and stretch over to the right in the same way. Breathe normally. ►Then, with your back straight, extend your spine forward. ►Relax down by breathing more deeply and bring your head to your knees. Close your eyes, holding for 10 seconds. Inhale and return to the start position. Repeat the exercise.

TRAVEL:
Hands and Feet

When you have to sit still for a long period while travelling on a plane, coach or train, your body stiffens up and you begin to feel lethargic and tired. Because you are in a confined space it is difficult to move and stretch your aching muscles without causing disturbance to the other passengers. This exercise will help to release any tension you may suffer in the sciatic nerves in your back and will also improve your blood circulation while you are forced to remain static. Gently moving your feet will alleviate any numbness or the 'pins and needles' that many people experience when they have to sit in a cramped position for any length of time.

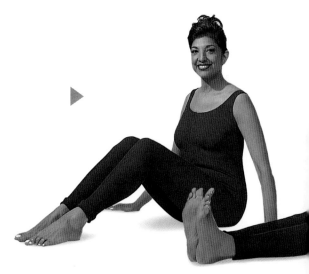

While you are seated, extend your legs forward and flex your toes upward. (If space is too limited to do this, you can perform the exercise in the normal sitting position.) ▶Point your toes and move both feet in a circle, first to the right and then to the left. ▶ Still pointing your toes, cross your ankles, roll onto your left hip and twist as far as you can. ▶Move back to the center and roll onto your right hip, twisting as far as you can. ▶Release your feet and sit up straight, taking your arms over your head with your elbows bent. Now shake your arms and hands to release any tension and improve your circulation. ▶Keep shaking both arms around your body until your hands come down to your hips. Repeat the exercise as necessary.

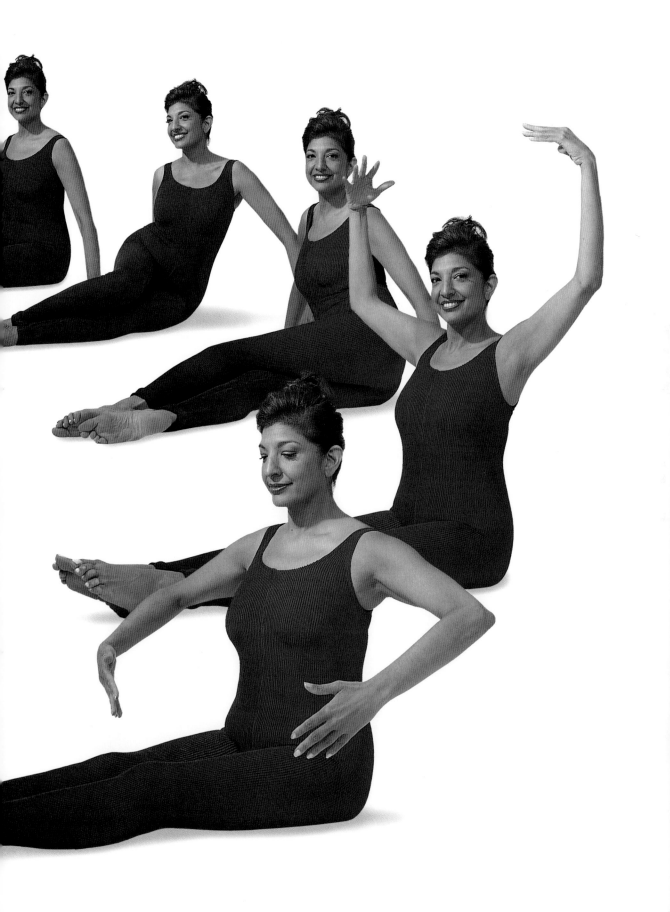

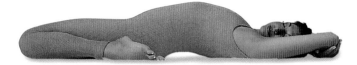

Art of Relaxation

Learning to soothe your nerves and calm your nervous system is the aim of the exercises in this chapter. Stress gets locked in the physical body and the goal is to release this muscular tension gently through a series of flowing movements. Stress can cause stiffness, especially in the neck, shoulders and lower back, leading to bad posture. Tension and stress are held in the body unconsciously and the moment people are made aware of their physical condition they will instinctively try to relax and find balance, as this is the natural state. Yoga is ideal for relaxation because it teaches you to shut yourself off from the rest of the world and go into the deeper realms of your mind to find lasting inner peace. When you relax deeply your nerve endings are rejuvenated and your nervous system functions better. The purpose of the exercises in the first part of this chapter is to release tension in specific muscle groups. The inverted postures, such as the modified shoulder stand, will calm the nervous system. Whenever the head drops forward, as in the forward stretch, a sudden feeling of calm will prevail. In the dead man's pose your body metabolism slows down. Make sure you are in a warm, quiet room wearing unrestricted clothing when you exercise. By doing these exercises you will bring peace to your body and mind at will.

Shoulder Shrugs and Rolls ▶

When people are very stressed and wound up, tension accumulates in the body, especially in the neck and shoulders. The only way to release this stiffness is to exaggerate the movement between the neck and shoulders while breathing deeply and evenly. When you do this exercise it is very important to keep your head straight and in correct alignment to your back and neck. As you inhale, focus your attention on the stiffness in your muscles and when you exhale imagine all the muscular tension leaving your body. Every person is different and will hold tension in certain weak spots. Visualize and concentrate on these areas and you will be amazed at how quickly you can feel relaxed.

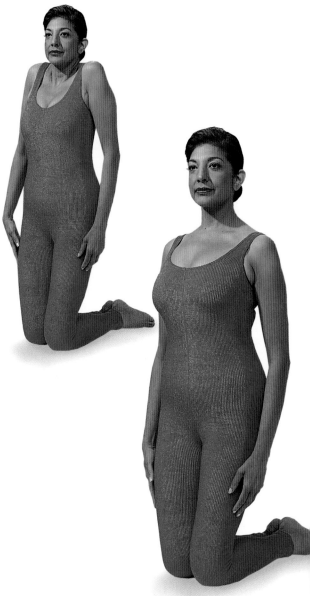

Kneeling on the floor, inhale and take your shoulders up high toward your ears. ▶As you exhale drop your shoulders down and push your shoulders blades together, opening out your chest. Repeat a few times until the stiffness starts to leave your body. Breathe deeply to help shift the tightness. ▶Now inhale and repeat the shoulder shrug. ▶As you exhale, move your shoulders back in a circular motion. ▶To repeat the exercise, inhale and take your shoulders forward and up, then exhale taking them back and down. Keep all your movements fluid and graceful. Return to the start position. As you exercise, keep still, concentrating on your neck and shoulders.

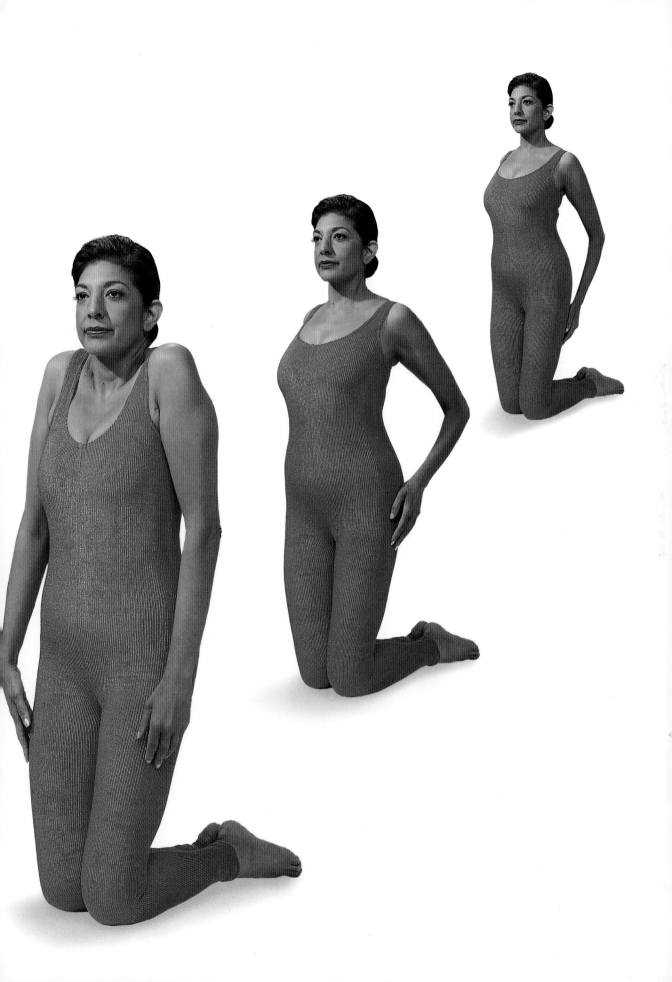

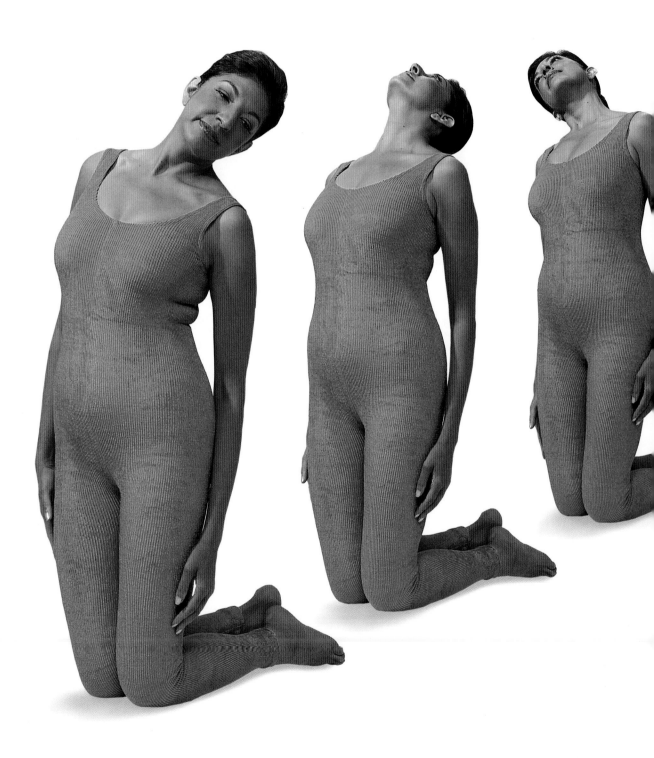

Head Rolls

These head rolls help to release tension not only in the neck and shoulders but also in the upper and middle section of the back. By keeping your upper body stationary you allow your head to move freely in all directions without any restrictions. Some people who have a lot of stress locked in the top area of their body experience pain as they rotate their head. If you feel a sharp pain stop at once, but most probably you will experience only a dull pain. When you feel any discomfort, stop in that position and breathe deeply through the pain until it passes. This exercise helps to release the congestion of twisted nerves and tight muscles by allowing the natural weight of the head to rotate evenly in all directions, alleviating the stress. Roll your head round carefully, keep your shoulder blades down at all times to maximize the stretch and concentrate on breathing deeply and evenly.

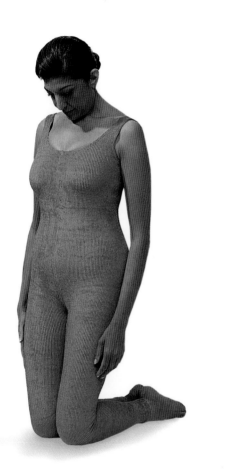

*For perfect posture
see page 32.*

Kneeling or sitting tall in perfect posture, begin the head rolls with your head in correct alignment to your neck and back. Drop your chin down onto your chest. ▶Inhale deeply and slowly roll your head in a circular pattern to your right shoulder. ▶Continuing to inhale, drop your head all the way back as far as possible without moving your shoulders and upper body. ▶Slowly exhale and take your head toward your left shoulder, then slowly bring your chin back down to your chest. Repeat the head roll clockwise and then two more times anticlockwise.

First Easy Warm-Up ▶

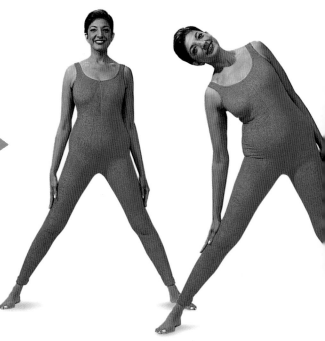

Stretching your body is the best way to release tension in all the muscle groups. Unless this stiffness is removed from your body the energy is blocked and cannot flow freely through your system. In yoga we stretch the muscles lengthwise while breathing correctly to produce a well-toned and invigorated body. As you bend and twist you free blockages, making your body more flexible, supple and relaxed. But remember not to force yourself – yoga is a gentle flow of movement. So begin slowly and do not be discouraged if at first your movements seem restricted. With practice you will experience great changes in your body and your attitude toward life.

Begin the warm-up standing with your legs 1–1.2m (3–4ft) apart and your toes pointing forward. Put your arms at your side and stand in perfect posture. ▶Inhale and gently lean to the right, keeping your spine straight in perfect alignment to your neck and head. Exhale and hold as you deepen your breath. ▶Inhale again and let your body weight stretch you sideways even further. Exhale, breathe normally, and feel the stretch from the left foot down to your right hand. Hold for 5 to 10 seconds. ▶Take your right hand toward your left leg and begin to twist your spine. ▶Inhale deeply and clasp your right hand to your left ankle and twist fully around. Exhale, but breathe deeply as you look over your left shoulder. Hold for 10 seconds. Release and return to the start position. Repeat on the other side.

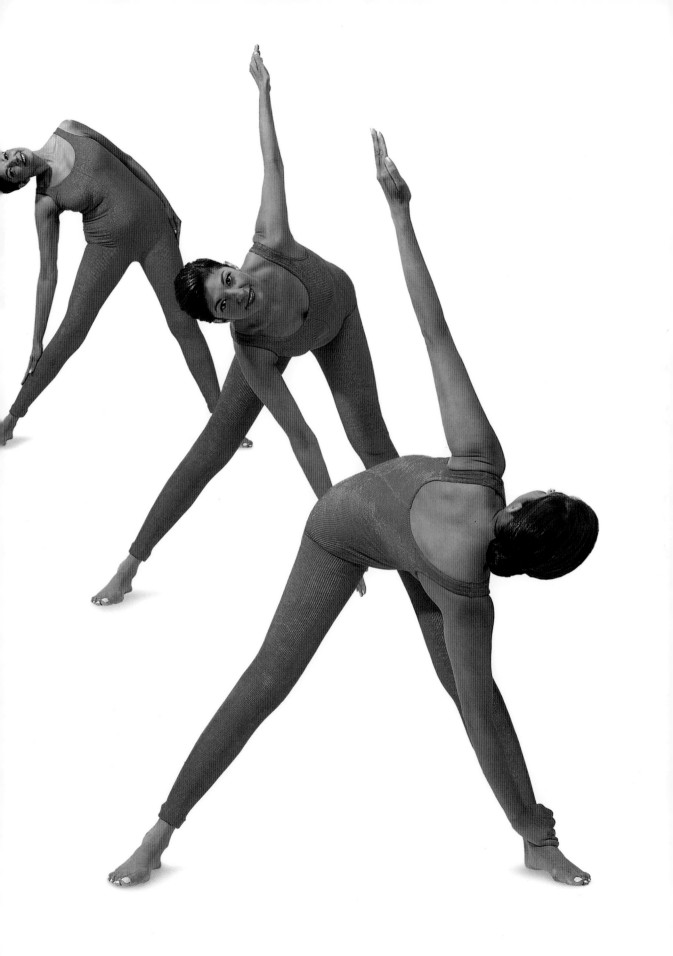

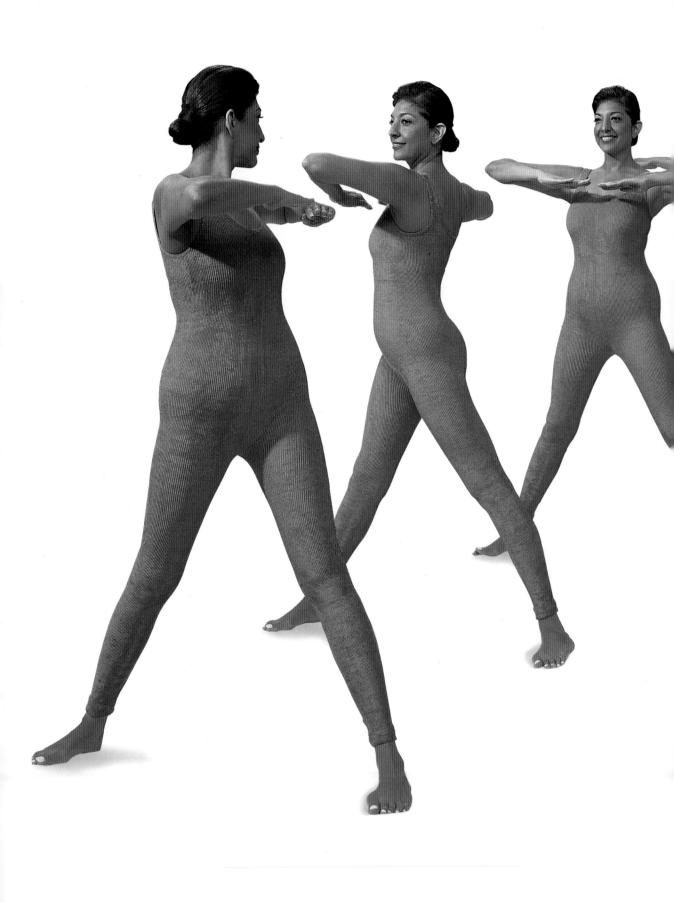

Second Easy Warm-Up

Twisting your body from side to side releases tension in the upper and lower back as well as in the hips and legs. It is important to keep the lower body stationary so that you can twist freely from the waist. It is a simple movement but has excellent effects because it helps to release toxins and tones the spine while stretching the backs of your legs. Make sure you keep your head upright in line with your spine. Your hips might have a tendency to sway but resist this movement by digging your heels down firmly into the floor and gripping hard with your toes.

Stand tall with your legs 1–1.2m (3–4ft) apart. Keep your toes pointing forward and stretch your arms out to the sides with your palms facing down. ▶Bend your elbows and keep your arms level to your chest. Make sure your shoulder blades are down. ▶Inhale and turn your upper body to the right, looking over your left shoulder. Exhale, inhale and turn your head to look over your right shoulder. ▶Bring your arms back to the front and twist around to the left side, looking over your right shoulder. Exhale, inhale and turn your head to look over the left shoulder. Repeat the whole exercise at least 5 to 10 times.

Back Roll ▶

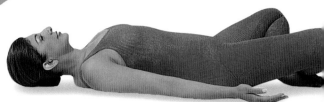

When you really need to relax this back roll releases any stress and strain from the tail-bone of the spine right up to the top of the neck. By taking your legs over your head you calm the nervous system and soothe the nerves. If you suffer from backache this is the easiest and safest exercise to relieve any pain. Also, when your body is feeling exhausted and needs a quick boost, this exercise combined with some deep breathing rejuvenates your entire system. You may find it hard in the beginning to take your legs right over your head, but just let the force of your natural body weight allow your legs and spine to roll over gently. At first you may need to push your palms down to the floor to help you roll over, but with practice you will soon realize that a supple spine is the main key to success.

Lie down on the floor with legs outstretched and arms at your side. Breathe deeply and evenly and feel your whole body relaxing. Draw your feet back, cross your ankles and place your palms upward, keeping your eyes closed. ▶ Bring your knees toward your chest and hold onto your toes, keeping your elbows straight. ▶ Inhale and slowly bring your knees and thighs down to your chest. ▶ Pull your tummy muscles in and start to take your legs over your head. ▶ Roll over completely and stretch your spine as far as possible. Keep your knees as close to your ears as possible and relax your neck and shoulder muscles. Exhale, and breathe deeply in this position, holding for at least 30 seconds. Repeat the exercise a few times until your body feels totally calm and relaxed.

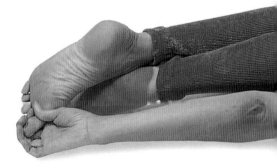

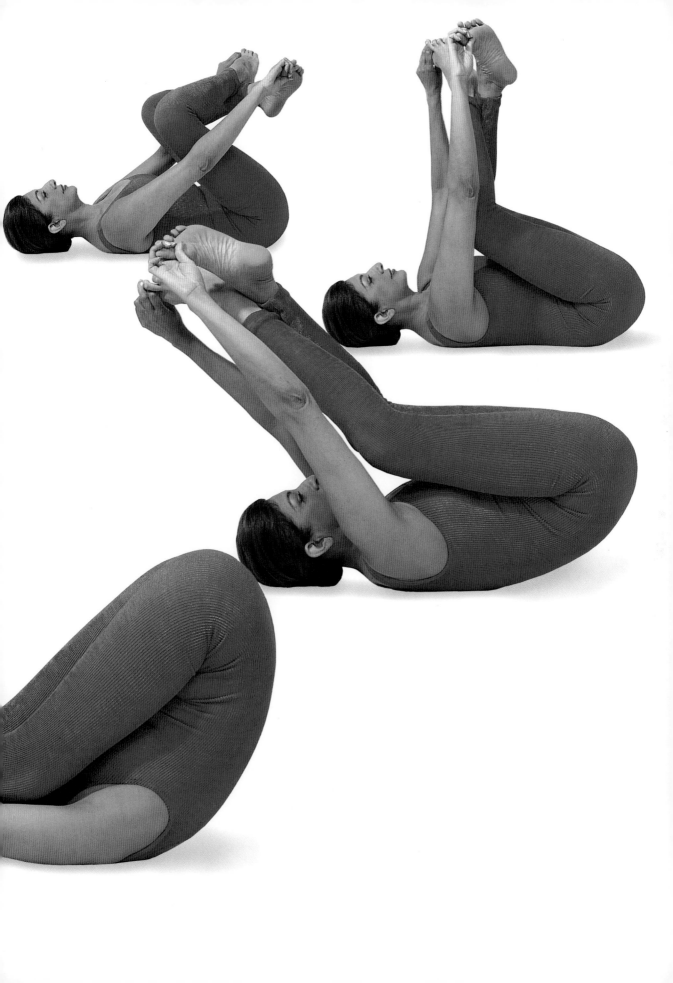

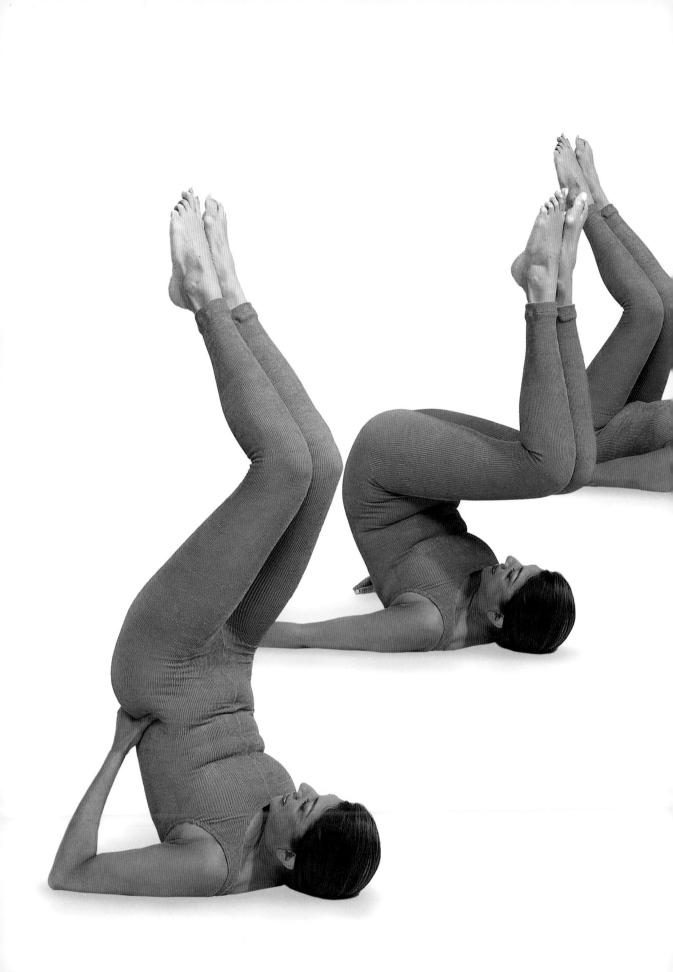

Modified Shoulder Stand

The shoulder stand helps to regulate your metabolism and balance your hormones. People who suffer regularly from stress often experience mood swings and weight fluctuations. This exercise helps to stabilize your temperament and weight and calms your mind. Two of the most important glands in the body are the pituitary and thyroid. According to the yogic texts, locking your chin into your chest stimulates your thyroid gland to help it function normally. When you are inverted with your legs above your head the blood flows downward to all your organs, replenishing and oxygenating the cells. This increased blood flow rejuvenates and relaxes your whole body.

Lie on the floor, legs outstretched and arms at your side. Bring your knees up, put your feet on the floor and place your palms facing down. ▸Inhale deeply, pushing your palms down, while bringing your knees up to your chest. ▸ Keep pushing your palms down and lift your spine off the floor. ▸ Take your hands to your waist to support your back and lift your legs up. Lock your chin into your chest. Exhale, and breathe normally while holding this position. Try to hold still for 30 to 60 seconds. To come down, inhale, and while exhaling slowly lower your back and legs to the floor. Keep breathing deeply and evenly. If you have any back discomfort do the back roll (see pages 66–67).

Knee Twist

This simple knee twist exercise helps to strengthen the spine as well as releasing toxins from the system. The more flexible your spine is, the more you will be able to twist around. It is very important to sit upright to lift your spine correctly. Some people who have weak backs might feel a dull pain in the lumbar region. As you build up these muscles you will feel uncomfortable if you are not sitting upright. The intensity of the twist is felt when the spine is the only part of the body that is moving as the hips stay immobile and in line. The most wonderful thing about twists is that there is no final position. Challenge yourself and try to twist even further every time you do this exercise.

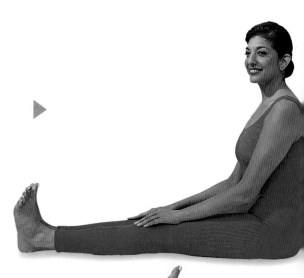

Start the twist sitting on the floor with your legs outstretched in front of you. Sitting up as tall as possible, flex your feet upward. ▶Bend your left knee and bring your foot in as close as possible, holding onto your leg with both hands. Make sure you do not collapse your spine at this time. If you feel your back caving in, place your foot further out. ▶With your right arm, hold onto your left leg with your right elbow in front of your knee for a tighter grip. ▶Take your left hand and place it on your lower back with your palm facing up. Inhale and twist as far as possible, looking over your left shoulder. Exhale and breathe normally as you deepen the twist. To release the spine, gradually unwind and return to the front, still holding your leg, and then return to the start position. Repeat the exercise on the other side, and then do twice on each side.

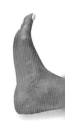

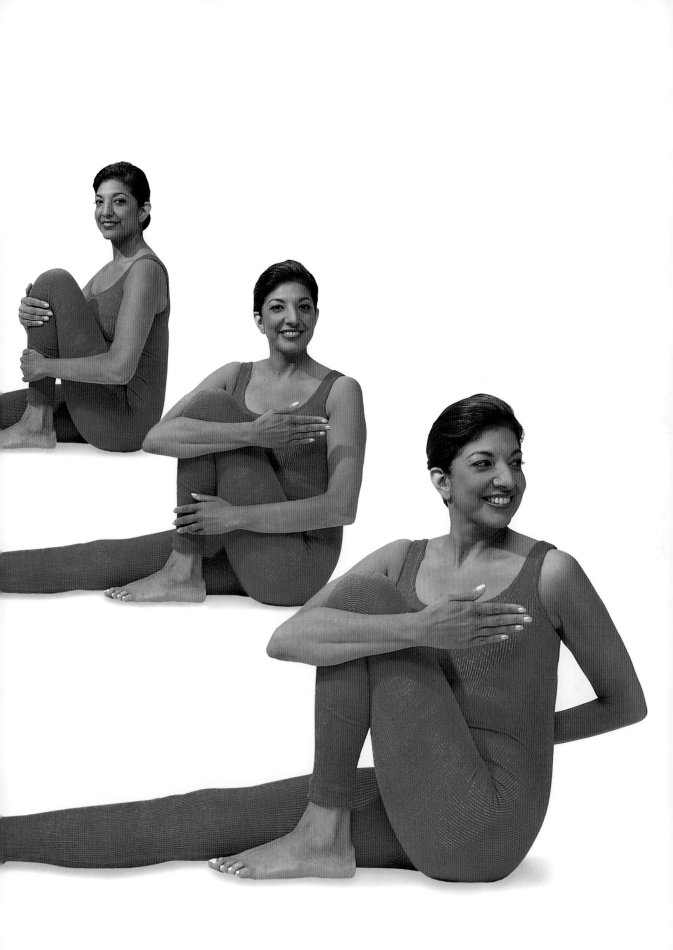

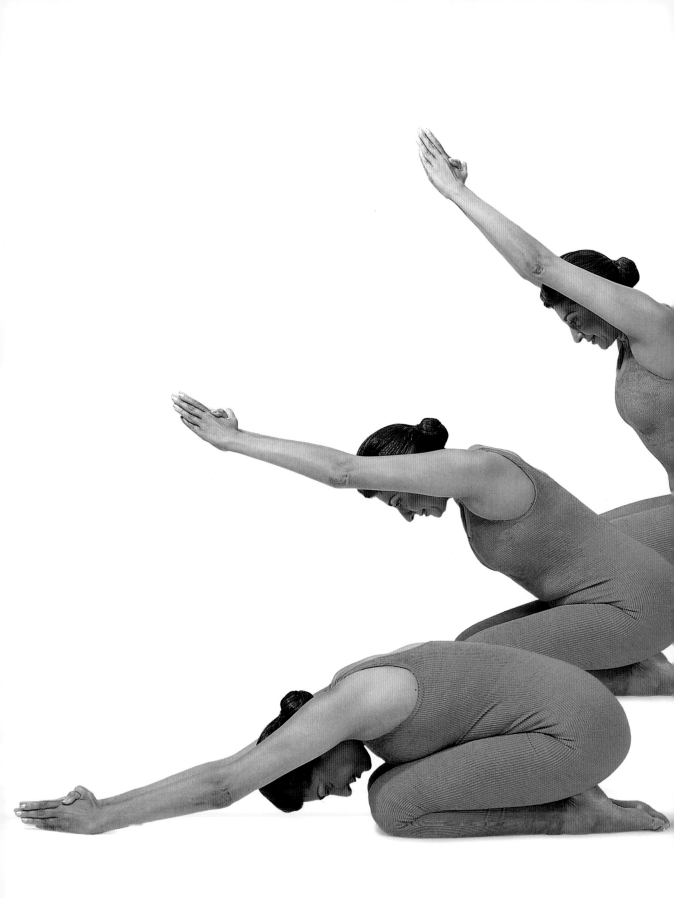

Forward Stretch

Stretching forward from the base of the spine helps to relax your brain and also soothes your nerves. The difficult part of this exercise is to keep your arms close to your ears and in line with your head as you lean forward. The tendency is to drop your head forward and to curve your spine. Stretch fully from the tailbone and tighten your abdominal muscles as you move forward. This pose looks like a simple exercise but it achieves many different, simultaneous effects: suppleness of the spine, more muscular strength, and also a deep relaxation that affects every part of the mind.

Start the exercise by kneeling down on the floor and stretching your arms straight above your head. Try to keep your elbows straight while keeping your palms together. As you stretch upward push your shoulder blades down and keep your arms as close to your ears as possible. ▶Inhale deeply and begin to stretch forward. Pull the tummy muscles in and keep your hips down toward your bottom. ▶ Continue to stretch forward with a straight spine. ▶Exhale and push your hands forward in front of you on the floor. Tuck your head in, pushing your face toward the floor. Breathe deeply and evenly and hold the position for at least 30 seconds, then slowly return to the start position.

Dead Man's Pose ▶

Relaxing is a technique that needs to be learned in order to maximize your capability for relaxation at will. Yoga is ideal because it allows your mind to shut out useless thoughts and relax the brain at a deeper level. This achieves stillness of the mind which helps to clarify thoughts and emotions. This exercise can rejuvenate your energy by relaxing every body nerve, and it can help cure insomnia. Find a quiet place and, because your body temperature drops, make sure you feel warm and comfortable.

Lie flat on the floor, knees up and arms at your side. If you wish to, you can put a small pillow under your head. Breathe deeply and evenly through your nose, mouth closed. Relax your face until you feel calm. ▶Slowly relax your legs down onto the floor. ▶Sink your tailbone into the floor, taking your arms out at your sides with palms facing upward. Leave your feet apart and your throat open. Keep breathing deeply and slowly. Now concentrate on each muscle group, beginning with the tummy, buttocks, thighs, knees, ankles, feet and toes. Inhale and tighten each section. Hold for 5 seconds. Exhale and release. Then work on the back, arms and hands. Tighten your fists to release tension. Now do your neck. Inhale, taking your shoulders up to your ears. Exhale and release. Repeat. Take your head from side to side and then let it drop. Relax your face. Keep still for 5 to 15 minutes. ▶To release, turn to one side, bringing your knees into your chest. Rest until you feel like getting up.

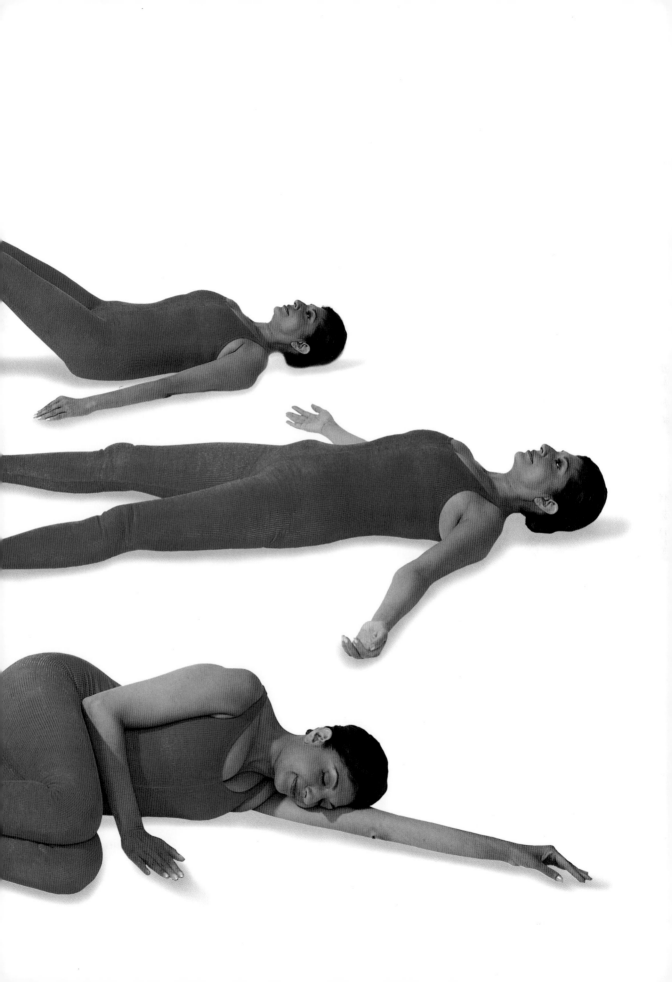

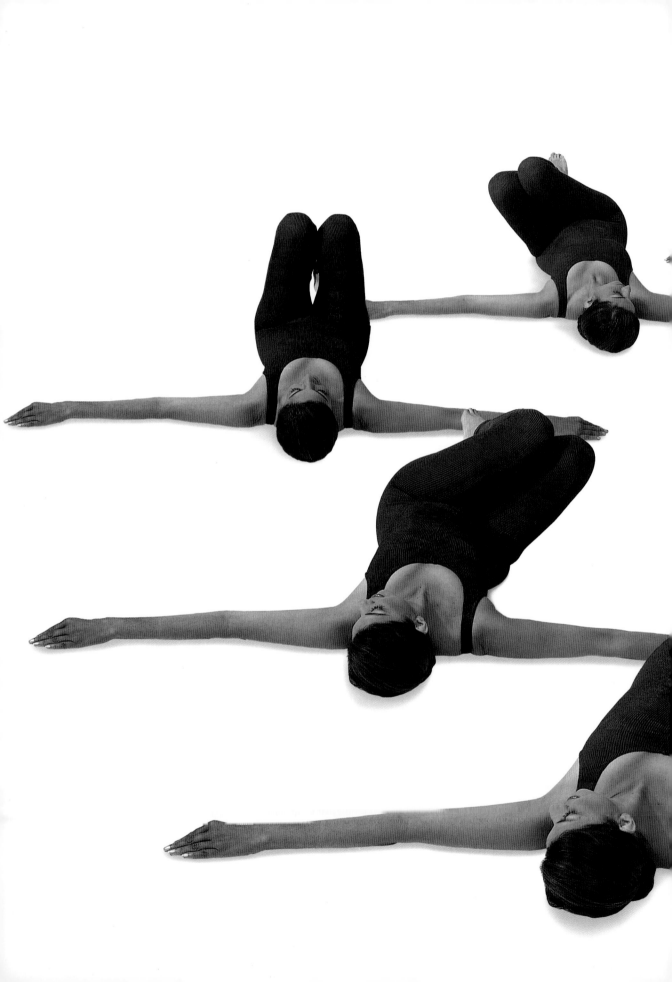

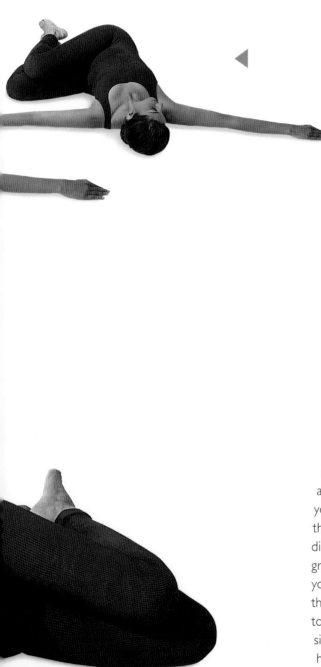

HOME:
Knee Twists

These simple knee twists are excellent to release tension throughout the body. As you ease your hips from side to side you can sometimes feel the muscles click into place to realign the spine. The movement also gives relief for backache. The blood supply to the discs and nerves is boosted, and the spine becomes toned. To twist laterally with safety, the pelvis should be the only region that moves; twisting from the shoulders and ribs can strain the lower back. Keep the movement graceful and fluid and use the tummy muscles to help control the action of twisting from one side to the other.

Start the exercise lying flat on the floor with your legs outstretched and your arms at your sides. Inhale and bring your knees toward your chest, stretching your arms to the sides with palms facing downward in line with the shoulders, as in position 3. Exhale and keep your neck and head in line with your spine. Inhale and as you exhale take your knees down to the floor on the left, while twisting your head in the opposite direction. ▶Inhale and bring your knees and head gradually back to the center. ▶Exhale and take your head to the left as you twist your knees to the right. Inhale and return your knees and head to the center. Exhale. Repeat the exercise from side to side until you feel that all your tension has been released and you are totally relaxed. Return to dead man's pose position 3 and 4 (see pages 74–75).

OFFICE:
Eyes, Jaw and Neck

Though space is limited in the office, it is still important to release any stress that builds up during the day due to the pressures at work. The first tension spots are the eyes, jaw, neck and shoulders, and this exercise is the most effective way of releasing all the stiffness in these areas quickly. You will feel relieved immediately and be able to face the rest of the day knowing that you have an instant solution if the problem reoccurs. During the exercise, breathe as deeply as possible to help movement and calm the nervous system.

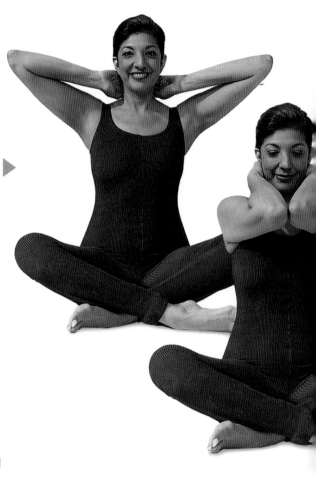

Sit on a chair or on the floor and cross your legs at the ankles. Sit up tall and clasp your hands behind your neck. Open out your elbows in line with your shoulders and push your shoulder blades down. ▶ Inhale deeply and slowly bring your elbows together. Exhale and return your elbows to position 1. Remember to keep your head straight in line with your neck and shoulders. Repeat. ▶ Now look upward as high as possible without tilting backward. Inhale, and bring your elbows together as before. Drop your head back and as you exhale open the elbows as much as possible. Open your mouth to release your jaw, and close. Repeat this jaw action twice and return to position 1. Repeat this section. Now release your arms and continue to sit upright. ▶ Rub your hands together to generate heat and blow into your palms. ▶ Place both palms over your eyes. This soothes the eyes and helps reduce pounding headaches. Breathe deeply and hold for as long as you can.

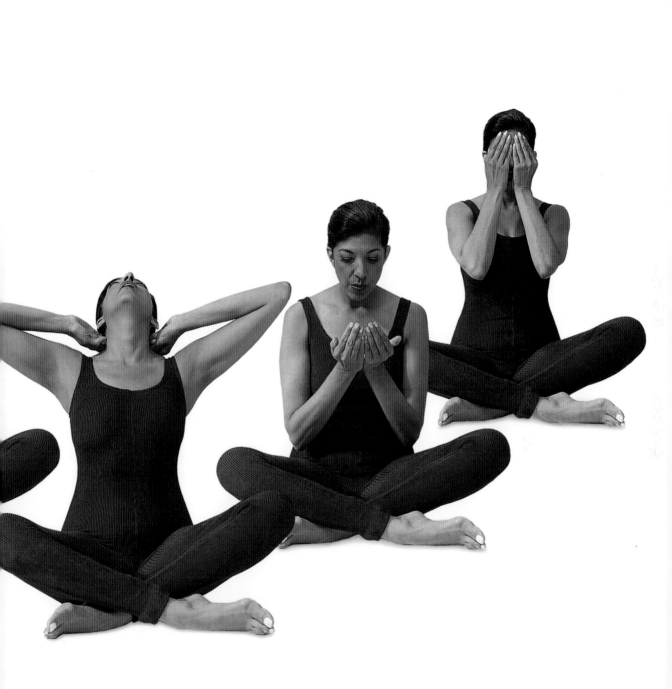

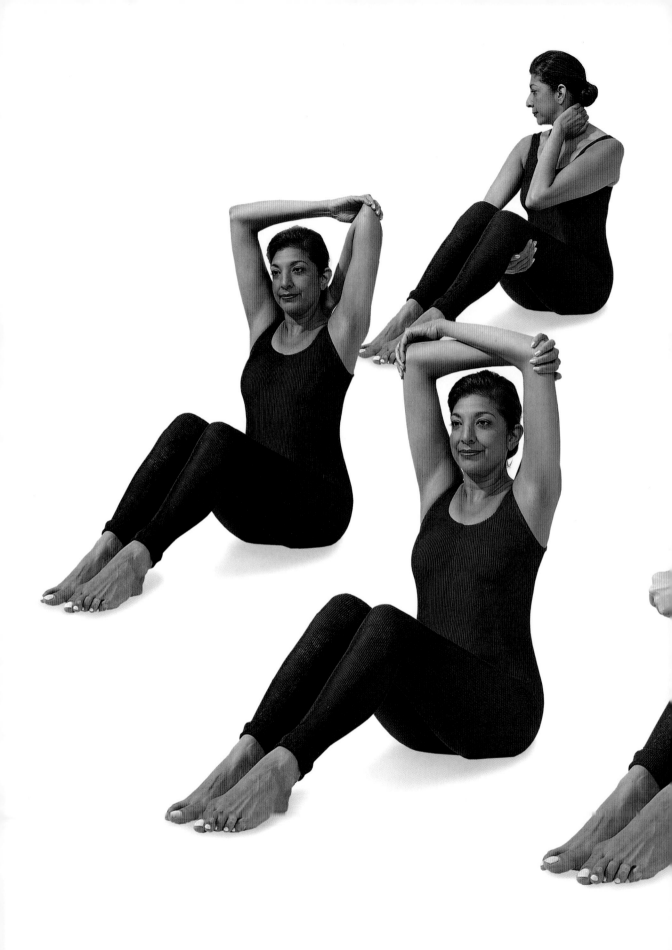

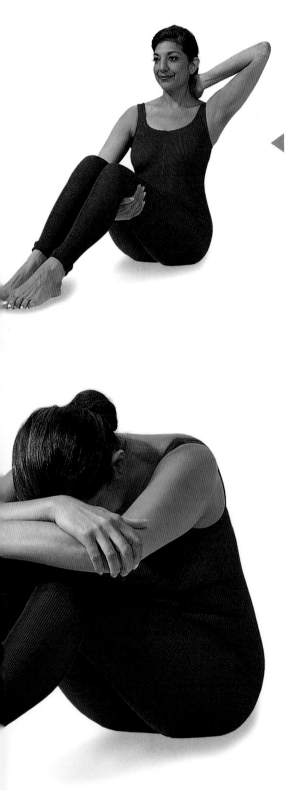

TRAVEL:
Hands and Feet

Whenever you sit still in one place for a length of time, as happens in travelling, your circulation becomes blocked. Also, some people feel panicky when they are confined to a small place where they cannot move around freely, and indeed many people have a real fear of travelling. Trying to keep calm and relaxed is the best solution to these insecurities. Breathing from your diaphragm acts as a natural tranquillizer to your nervous system, so the deeper you breathe the calmer your mind will become. During these stress-ful travel situations, start to lengthen your breaths and soon you will be taking deep breaths naturally.

Start by sitting upright in your plane or train seat or when you are taking a break from driving. Take your left hand around the back of your neck and open out your elbow. ▶Inhale and twist your neck and head to the right, bringing your elbow down into your chest to increase the stretch. Exhale, and return to position 1. Repeat 2 to 3 times. Now take your right hand around the back of the neck and repeat the exercise 2 to 3 times. ▶Return to position 1 and take your right hand to hold your elbow behind your head. Stretch both elbows back. Breathe normally, and repeat on the other side. ▶ Now clasp both elbows with your hands over your head and take them back behind your ears. Breathe normally and hold for 5 to 10 seconds. ▶Relax forward, placing your forehead down on your knees or table. Relax deeply, breathing evenly, and feel the stress leave your spine.

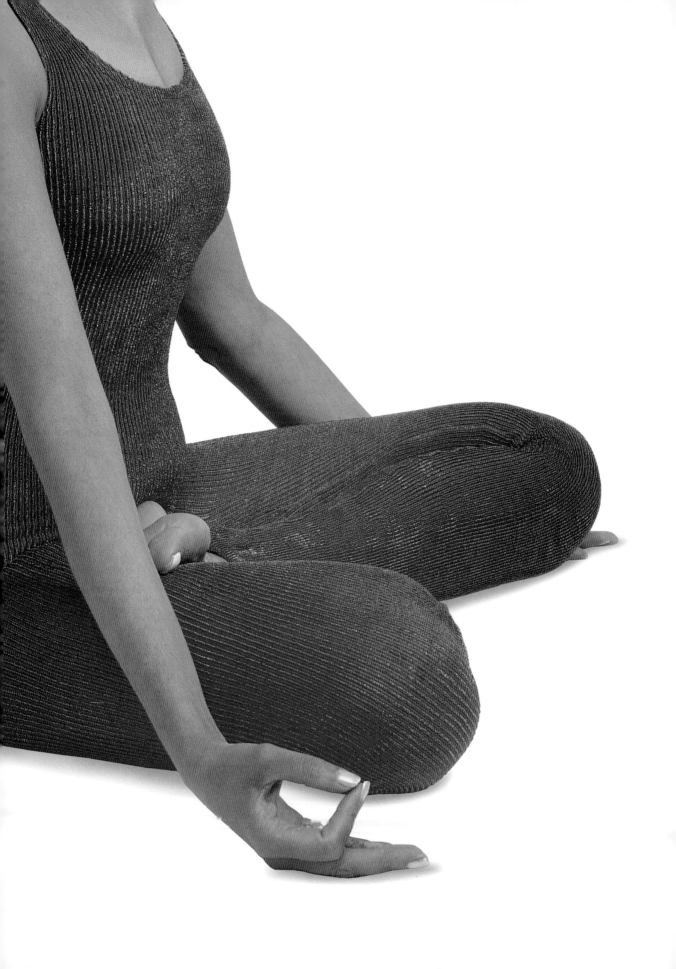

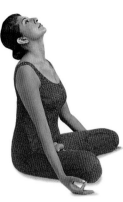

Meditation and Visualization

Meditation is a skill that clarifies and focuses the mind. Mastery over the mind is achieved through yoga meditation because it teaches you to concentrate on one subject in the first stage and calm your mind in the second. Mental breakdowns caused by stress can be greatly alleviated. Through meditation a person can observe their symptoms and reactions objectively, and change their attitudes toward their ailment. Meditating will bring them back to harmony and restore the balance that was lost. The yoga student can use meditation for practical purposes or move ahead into the deeper realms of the mind to discover universal truths and spiritual bliss. We begin with breathing exercises to calm the mind, as deep breathing acts as a natural tranquilizer. The meditation poses are all sitting positions to keep your spine erect. The true position is the lotus, because your tailbone nearly touches the floor, allowing the energy to move freely through the body's energy centers to the crown *chakra* (see page 90) in the head to connect with cosmic energy. Visualization is another technique to help train your mind for meditation. To start visualizing, sit in a meditation pose and think of a happy experience when you were close to nature. Observe your surroundings, emotions and reactions to the environment to stop your mind wandering.

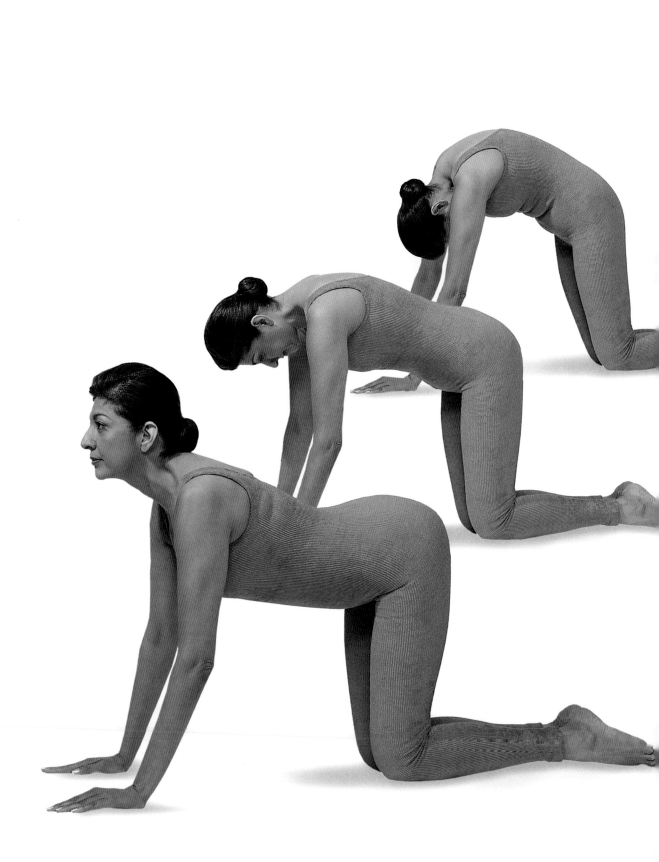

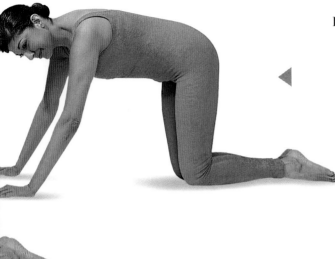

Breathing

Learning how to control your breathing is fundamental to training and controlling your mind. In this exercise we learn how to contract and release the abdominal muscles to regulate the flow of *prana*, or energy. Because of these movements the abdominal organs are toned and internally massaged and the gastric juices are stimulated, which aids digestion. The exercise helps to eliminate toxins in the digestive tract as well as regulating the bowel. The contraction and release action helps to trim excess fat from the stomach and flatten the tummy. It is always best to do this *bandha* or breathing technique on an empty stomach. Allow 4 to 6 hours after eating a heavy meal, but a light beverage such as tea can be taken 30 minutes before. The more you do this exercise, the more you will notice the benefits. At first you might find it difficult to regulate your breathing correctly, but with practice you will understand why this breathing technique is taught to maintain good body health.

Start the exercise kneeling on the floor with your hands directly in line with your knees. Inhale deeply and then exhale quickly through your nose so that air is forced from your lungs in a rush. ▶When all your breath is totally released, hold your breath and contract your abdominal muscles upward behind your rib cage toward your spine. Hold for 5 seconds. ▶Still holding your breath, release your muscles and rib cage. Hold for 5 seconds. ▶Inhale again and arch your spine down. Exhale and breathe normally. Repeat the whole exercise 2 times and build up to 10 times or more.

Pranayama
(bellow)

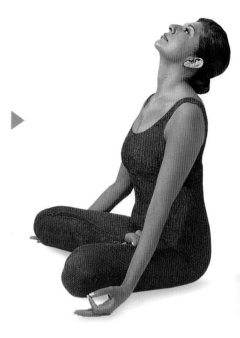

It is important to learn how to breathe properly, so set aside a regular time in a comfortable, airy space each day to practice *pranayama* techniques. *Pranayama* is the science of breath control. This particular breathing exercise is a simple one for beginners and helps you understand how to regulate your breathing pattern. At first you might find it difficult to lengthen your breath and exhale in a controlled way. Look at your posture, your breathing rhythm, and the way in which you breathe. When you exhale, your rib cage should expand forward and sideways, but the area below your shoulder blades and armpits should expand only forward. Note that the thumb and finger contact signifies the symbol of knowledge. The thumb is the universal soul and the index finger the individual soul; together they form the seal of wisdom.

Sit cross-legged, hands on the floor, with a straight spine and your head in line with your neck. Relax your muscles, especially in your face. Close your eyes to calm your mind. Breathe deeply and evenly. Take your thumb and index finger together. Inhale deeply through your nose and drop your head back without moving your spine. ▶Open your mouth slightly and form the letter 'O'. ▶Slowly exhale through your mouth as you drop your head until your chin rests on your chest. ▶Do not cave in your chest or spine, and exhale evenly. The longer you exhale the better, so when practiced, exhale for 5 seconds, building up to 10 seconds. Repeat at least 5 times.

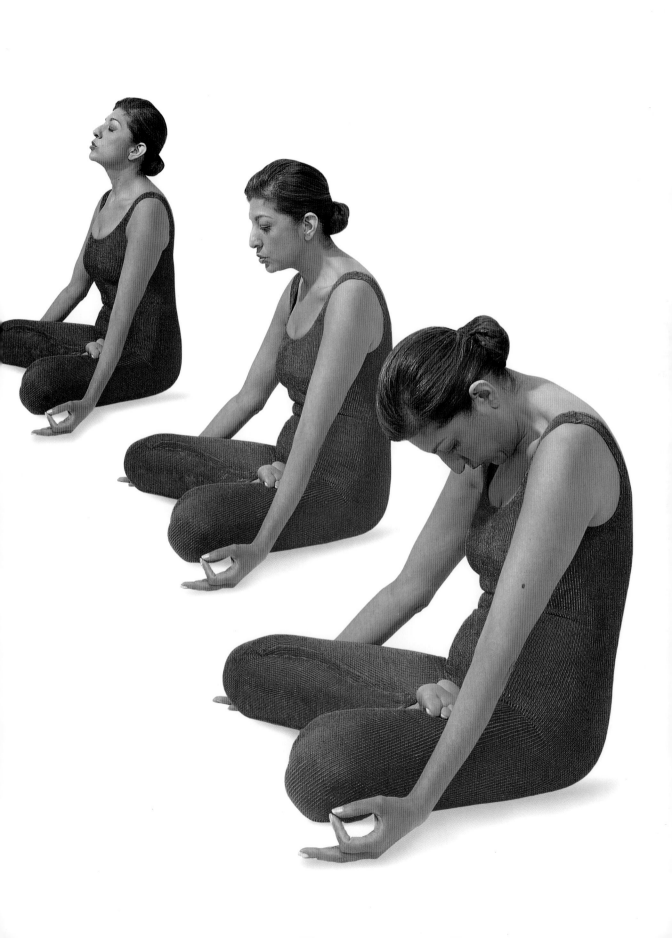

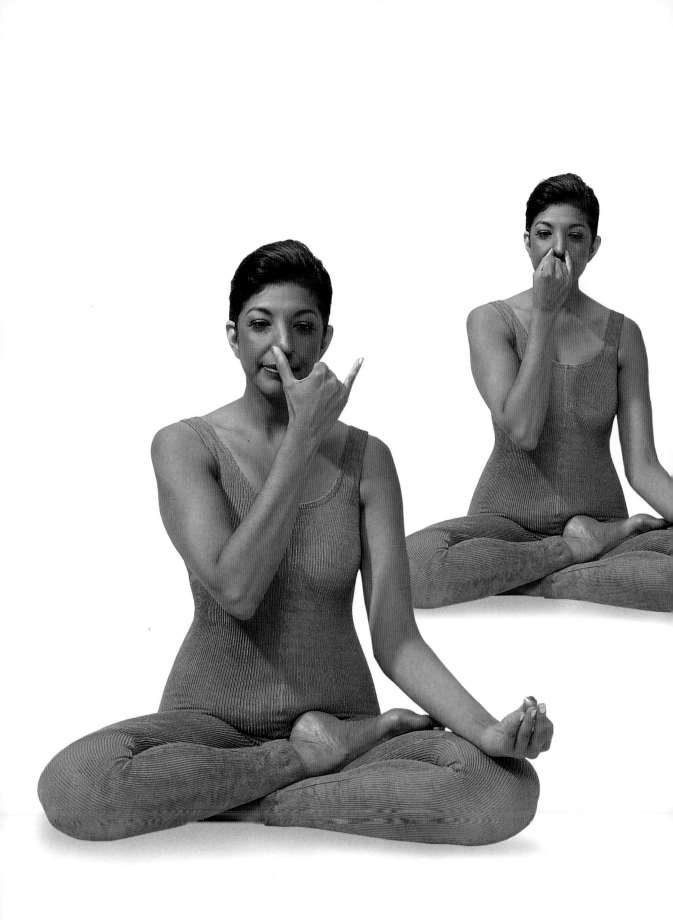

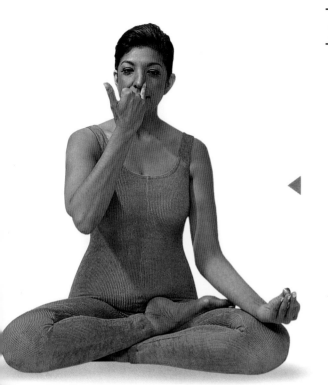

Pranayama
(nostril breathing)

Alternate nostril breathing is an advanced breathing technique. The energies of the body, whether male or female, have both masculine and feminine properties. The right side signifies the masculine energies, while the left side is the feminine. Alternate nostril breathing harmonizes these energies to restore balance to mind and body. The even breathing strengthens your nerves and encourages a balanced temperament and sound mind. Keep your breaths long, steady and deep. If you cannot maintain an even breathing rhythm, stop immediately in case you strain your lungs and diaphragm, and check your technique.

Sit crosslegged on the floor. Lift your spine up, but keep your shoulders down. Keep the thumb and index finger together on your left hand and rest it on your left knee. Bend your three main fingers into your right palm, but stretch up your thumb and little finger. Block your left nostril with your little finger and breathe deeply through your right nostril. Close your eyes, relaxing your face and body muscles. Inhale for 5 seconds and exhale for 5 seconds. Repeat 10 times on the right nostril and then block the right nostril with your thumb and repeat 10 times on the left.
▶Then inhale from the right for 5 seconds, hold your breath for 3, blocking your nostril with your thumb, and exhale through the left for 5 seconds. ▶ Inhale from the left nostril for 5 seconds, hold for 3, and exhale through the right for 5 seconds. Repeat the exercise at least 10 times.

Chakras and Candle Gazing

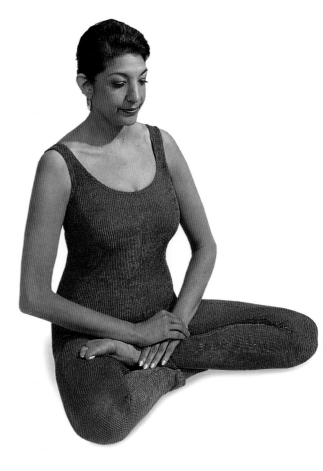

Chakra is a Sanskrit word meaning 'wheels' that radiate energy in a circular pattern through the spine's vital centers. Just as antennae pick up radio waves and turn them into sound, *chakras* pick up on cosmic vibrations and distribute them through the body's energy centers. To maintain good health it is vital to keep the centers generating equal energy through the body. If a *chakra* is blocked with too much or too little energy the body becomes unbalanced. Acupuncture uses needles placed in the energy centers to restore balance, and in yoga we learn *pranayama* (breath control) to ensure that the correct energy flows evenly through the body. Candle gazing (see page 93), a technique to train the mind to focus on one thought, helps to restore harmony to the mind and body by keeping the *chakras* balanced. There are seven *chakras.* The first is in the pelvic region and relates to the sexual organs and procreation. The second is in the belly button, controlling emotions. The third is in the solar plexus, ruling the stomach and digestive tract. The fourth is the heart *chakra,* which relates to love. The fifth, in the throat, relates to communication. The sixth is the third eye (the spot between the eyebrows) that rules higher consciousness. The seventh *chakra* is the crown *chakra,* uniting a person with the cosmic universe.

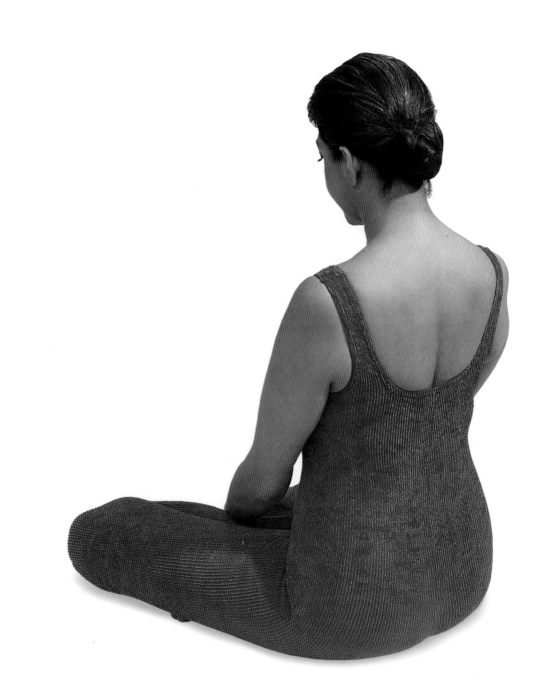

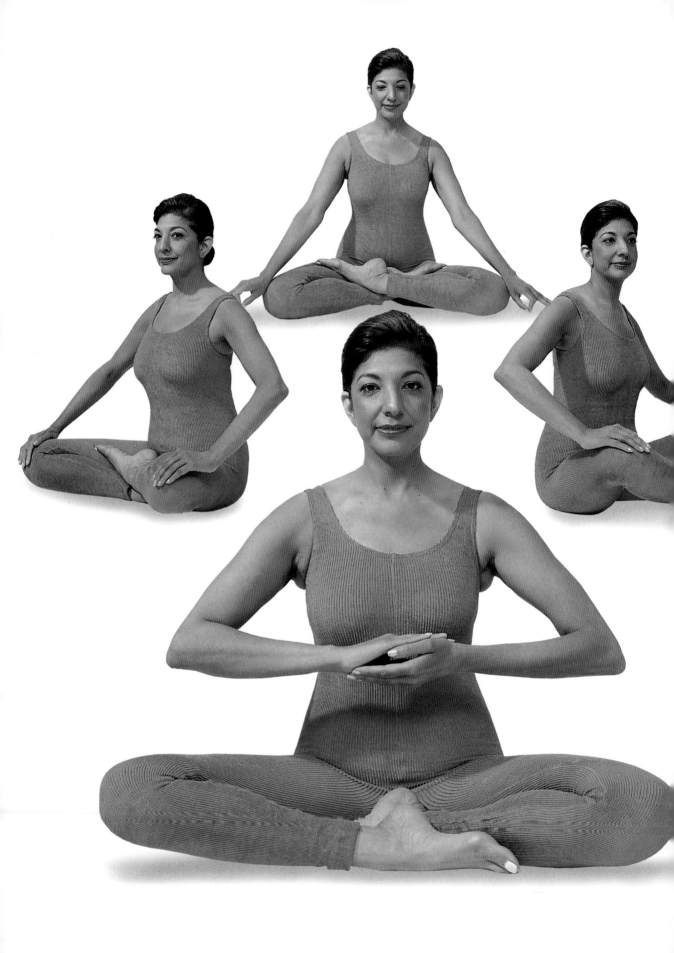

Meditation Poses

All meditation poses are sitting positions that vary only in how the legs are placed. Whether you are sitting cross-legged, in half-lotus or full lotus position, or with your heels together, your back must be erect from the base of your spine to your neck and be perpendicular to the floor. There should be no strain on the body. Keep your tongue still and your eyes closed. In meditation the brain is passive, but alert. If your organs are not functioning correctly the brain will send warning signals immediately. Meditation focuses the mind on one thought alone, and is useful to discipline and calm the mind. It is hard to sit still when your mind is wandering, but meditation teaches you how to shut yourself off from the world and find inner peace.

Meditation Poses

Top: Lotus
Left: Half-lotus
Right: Cross-legged
Bottom: Heels together

The first technique to learn is candle gazing. Place a candle in front of you so that the candle is in line with the point between your eyebrows. Now gaze at the candle and observe the flicker, the candle's size, and every aspect of it. After 30 to 60 seconds close your eyes. You will retain an optical image of the candle and the flicker of light in your mind. When the flicker starts to disappear, force the image to stay. This trains your mind to concentrate hard. At first it seems impossible to maintain the image but with continued practice it becomes easy. The next step is meditation. Focus your attention on the third eye and concentrate on one thought. Keep breathing deeply and notice your even breathing rhythm, while focusing your mind on one thought.

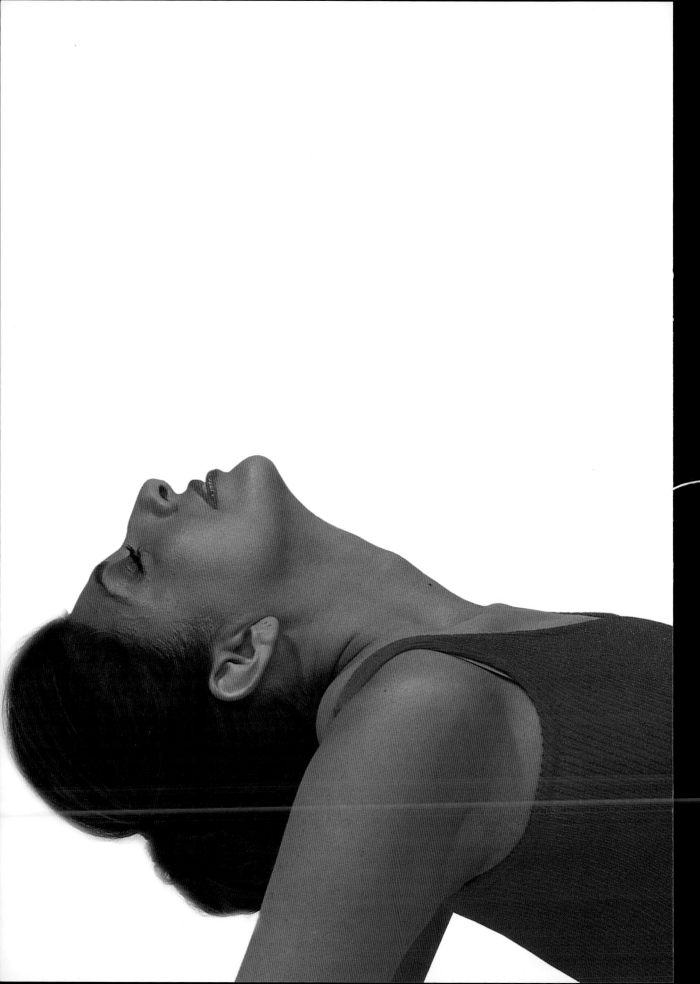

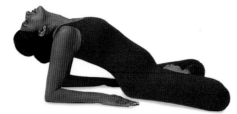

Remedial Yoga

Prana is the Sanskrit word for the energy that flows through the body. There are seven energy centers in the body and it is vital that energy flows freely through the system for good health. When people are stressed some centers become blocked, causing an imbalance. Yoga focuses on correct breathing techniques to increase the lung capacity and bring fresh oxygen to the vital organs. It is now possible to prove scientifically the effect of remedial yoga, and clinical trials have shown its beneficial results. There are four phases of stress disorders. The first is the psychic phase. There is irritability, energy loss, sleeplessness and anxiety attacks. If unchecked the person moves to the second, psychosomatic phase and experiences hypertension, tremors or palpitations. The next phase is the somatic phase when illness develops in the vital organs. The fourth phase is the organic phase when the affected organ is in full-fledged chronic inflammatory change. Medical attention is now required. Yoga can help prevent the first phase, relieve the symptoms in the second phase, develop a therapy programme in the third, and with modern medicine help the body return to its normal state in the fourth phase. Remedial yoga takes the stress disorder and applies a specific exercise that will alleviate the symptoms, or a series of exercises to help cure the ailment.

Here I have prescribed the *asana* specific to some common ailments. There are some that respond particularly well, such as asthma, migraine and digestive disorders.

HEAD:
Headaches

When your head is pounding because of tension and other mental anxieties, dropping your head forward relieves the pressure in no time. The blood rushes to the brain and soothes the nervous system. Many people find this uncomfortable at first and may even feel dizzy and nauseous. In fact, it will probably feel as if the pain is increasing rather than decreasing. But do not panic, just give yourself time to get used to this sensation. Just breathe deeply throughout the exercise and the pain and panic will soon subside. Make sure you keep your weight evenly distributed between your heels and toes to maintain your balance. Keep your movements fluid and try not to pause between positions.

Stand upright with your feet together in perfect posture. Inhale deeply and as you exhale drop your body forward. Bend your knees, relax your head and neck, shake out your arms and take your hands to the floor with your palms facing upward. Relax every muscle in your body. Hold for 30 seconds, breathing deeply. ▶Slowly inhale and lift your body slowly upward, still keeping your head and arms forward. ▶Now push your hips forward and drop your shoulders down. Then shift your weight to your heels, open out your chest and drop your head all the way back. Exhale, and breathe normally while you hold the position for 5 seconds. Lift up your head again and return to the start position. Repeat the whole exercise.

For perfect posture see page 32.

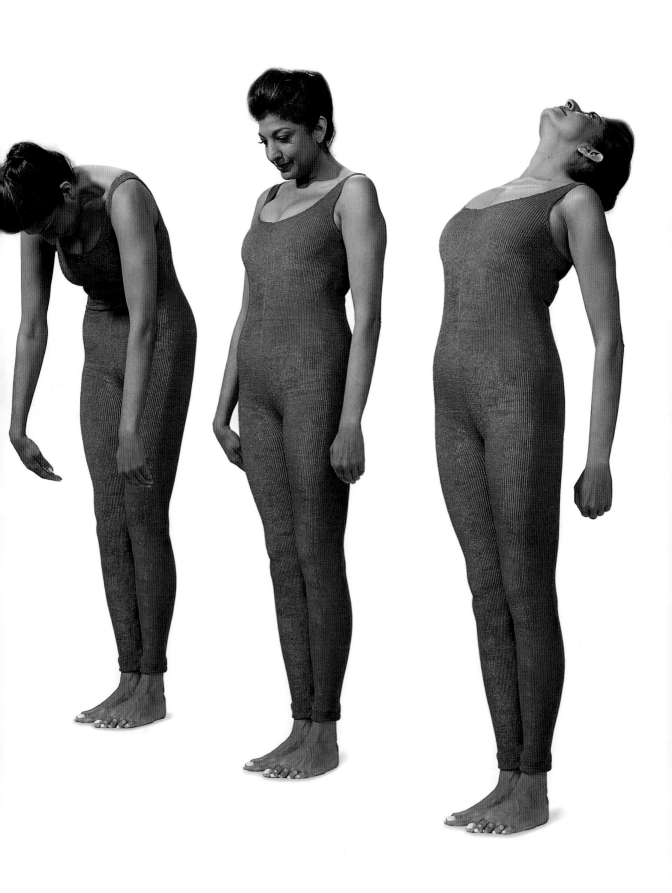

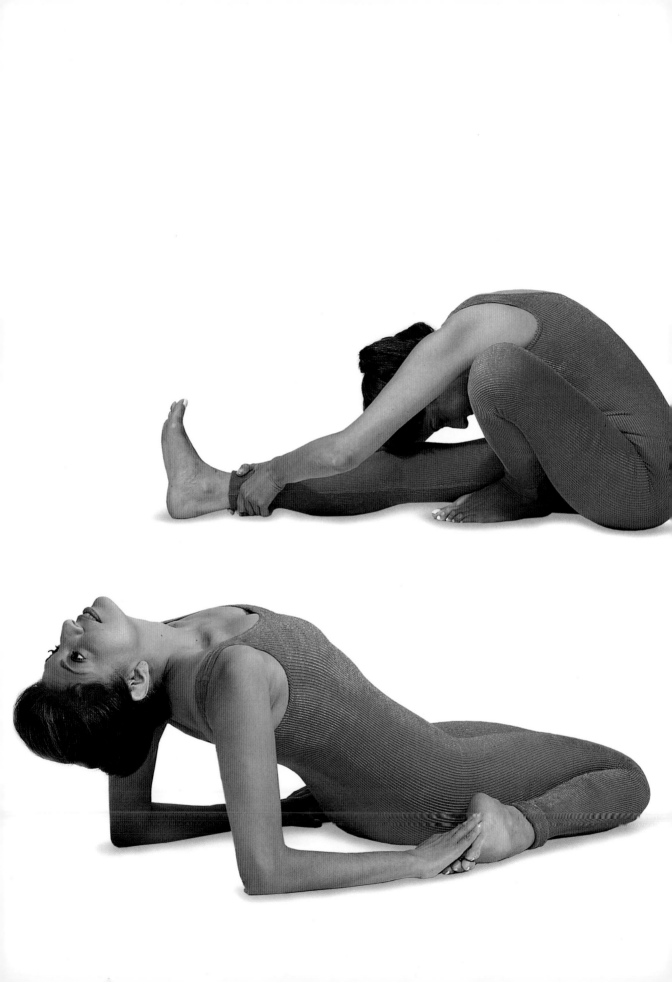

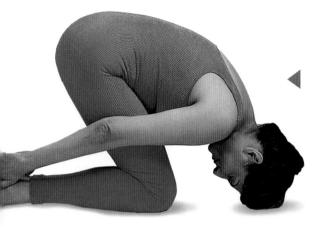

HEAD:
Brain

The brain is the seat of all intelligence, wisdom and discrimination. When you are affected by loss of memory or lack of sleep, these positions make pure blood flow through the brain cells, rejuvenating them so that thought processes become clearer. They are also a tonic for people whose brains tire easily. You cannot function well without a healthy brain so if stress affects it, take steps before problems such as migraine and insomnia set in.

This exercise is excellent for relieving headaches and stimulating the brain cells. Sit upright on both knees, spine straight. Clasp your hands to your ankles, or put your palms flat in front of you. Place your forehead on the floor. Inhale and roll forward on to the top of your head. Exhale, and release the neck stretch. Repeat 5 times.

To get the blood flowing, sit with legs stretched out in front. Flex your feet upward. Bring your left foot as high as possible toward your right thigh. Clasp your hands around your right ankle or leg. Inhale, pull your tummy muscles up and stretch forward, lengthening from your tailbone. Exhale, and drop your forehead to your right knee. Hold for 10 seconds, breathing deeply. Release and sit up. Change legs and repeat on the other side.

Another head exercise is to sit up with knees together. Inhale then exhale while you drop your head back and lean backward, supporting yourself on your elbows. Hold for 5 seconds, breathing normally. Release and repeat.

HEAD:
Mind

When people suffer from stress they can find it difficult to focus their mind for any length of time. Their thoughts are often confusing and conflicting. By doing balancing exercises you can help to focus your mind and improve your concentration. The concentration needed to stand on one leg can help you push distracting or negative thoughts from your mind. These exercises are quite challenging and at first you might think that you are incapable of balancing on one leg, but with perseverance you will soon reach your goal.

Stand up straight, feet together, in perfect posture. Breathe normally and draw your energies into yourself. Hold for 5 seconds. Place your right foot with your heel and toe in line with your left ankle. Place your palms together in front of your chest. Hold for 5 seconds. ▶With your right hand lift your right leg and place it on your inner left lower leg, knee, or inner thigh according to your flexibility so that your knee is at right angles to the straight leg. Palms together, take your arms over your head and balance. Hold for 5 to 10 seconds and focus on an object in front of you to aid concentration. Repeat on the other side.

The one leg balance (see right) is more difficult. Stand upright with feet together. Take both hands to the floor to balance, clasp your right ankle anywhere on your leg and focus on one spot on the floor in front of you. ▶Inhale, pull your tummy muscles in and lift your left leg up high without twisting your hips. Exhale and breathe normally. Repeat on the other side.

For perfect posture see page 32.

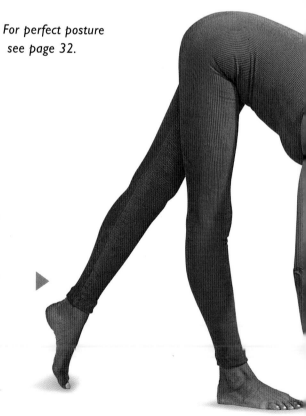

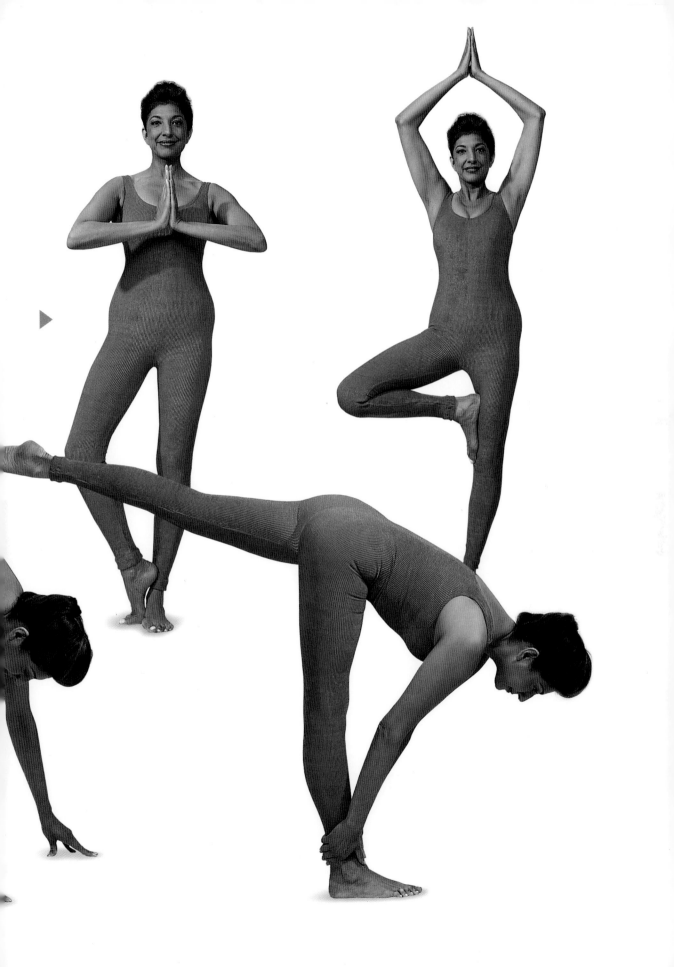

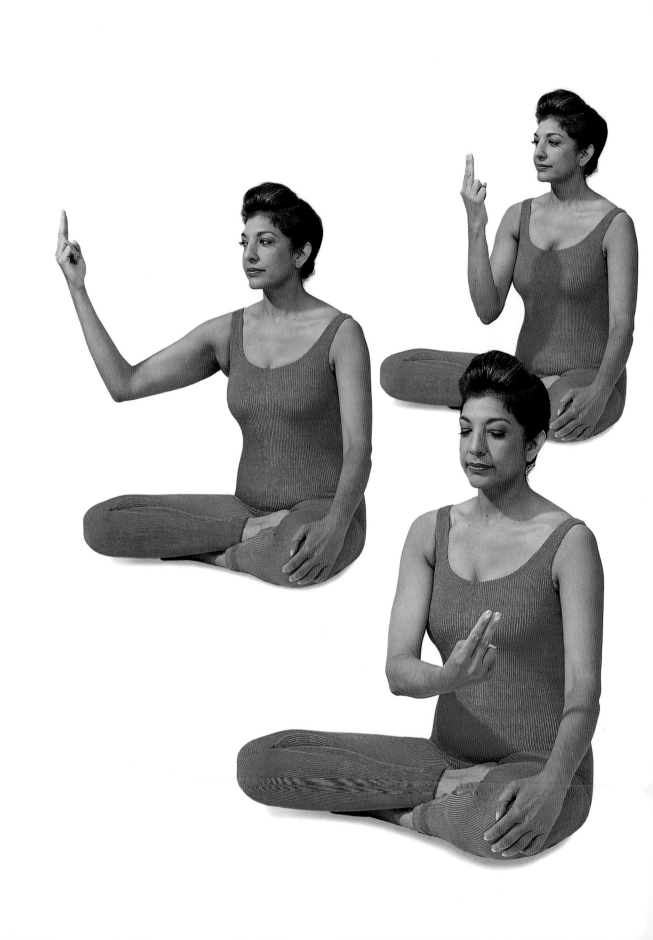

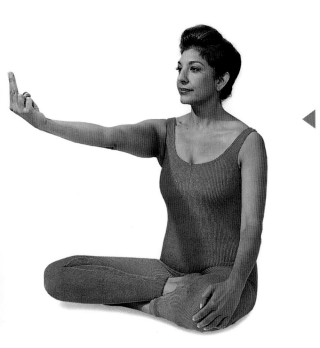

HEAD:
Eyestrain

When people are stressed and tired they complain about blurred vision and sore eyes. This exercise relieves eyestrain and strengthens the eye muscles. Many people neglect their eyes and forget that these muscles need to be toned. When you are doing these exercises keep your head and neck still – just move your eyes. Initially your eyes may hurt because the muscles are weak, but as you get used to these eye movements the muscles will strengthen and you will feel no strain. As we age these muscles weaken and most people need glasses to read or see properly. If you practice eye movements twice a day you will soon find a marked improvement in your eyesight.

Sit tall crosslegged on the floor. Rest your left palm on your left knee and straighten out your right arm in front of you. Curl your fingers into your palm, but straighten out the first two fingers. Take the fingers in front of your nose with a straight elbow and focus your mind on them. ▶ Slowly bring your fingers toward your nose. Do not be distracted from your focal point. Touch your fingers to your nose while turning your eyes inward. ▶ Hold for 5 seconds, and slowly extend your arm back to the first position. If your vision is blurred, force your eyes to focus clearly. Close your eyes to rest and repeat. ▶ Still sitting tall, take your fingers up high to the right. Draw an imaginary diagonal line from the top right-hand corner to the low left-hand corner. Do not turn your head. Change hands and repeat the entire exercise.

CIRCULATION:
Energy

People who are sluggish usually have poor circulation. They suffer from chronic fatigue because they are stressed and their muscles remain tense even when they are resting. The only way to reduce stress levels is to improve circulation, which will then alleviate depression and lack of energy. People with bad circulation always have cold hands and feet, even in the summer, and are more susceptible to colds and flu. To boost your energy, stretch and move gently in different directions. This exercise increases energy flow, while deepening your breathing and toning your body. Do not force your body, just try to increase flexibility and stamina.

▶

Stand tall with feet 1–1.2m (3–4ft) apart and toes pointing forward. Inhale, and throw your arms above your head with elbows straight and palms facing each other. Exhale and breathe normally. ▶ Simultaneously, turn your right foot and body to the right. Turn your left foot, so that the instep is in line with your right heel, keeping your hips and shoulders square and your arms close to your ears. ▶ Inhale and lunge forward with your right knee. Exhale. Keep your spine erect and your back leg and knee straight. Breathe deeply and hold for 5 seconds. ▶ Inhale, straighten your right leg and as you exhale, lean forward, arms outstretched, with a flat back. Cross your thumbs, with palms together. ▶ Inhale and bend your right knee, stretching your arms out further. Push your left foot firmly down to help your balance. Exhale, deepen your breath and hold for 10 to 15 seconds. Repeat the exercise with the other leg.

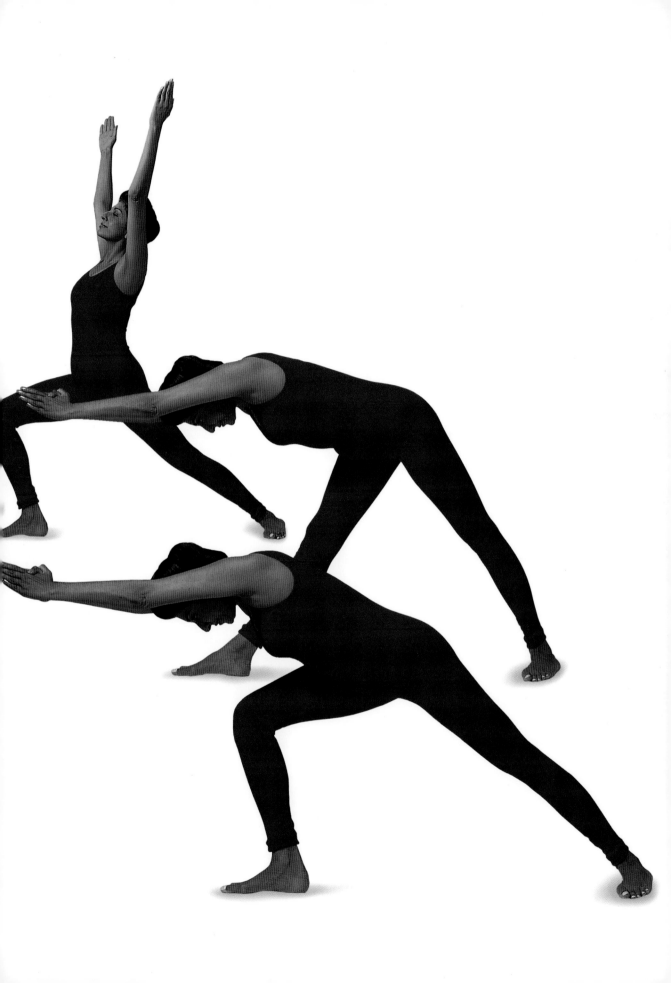

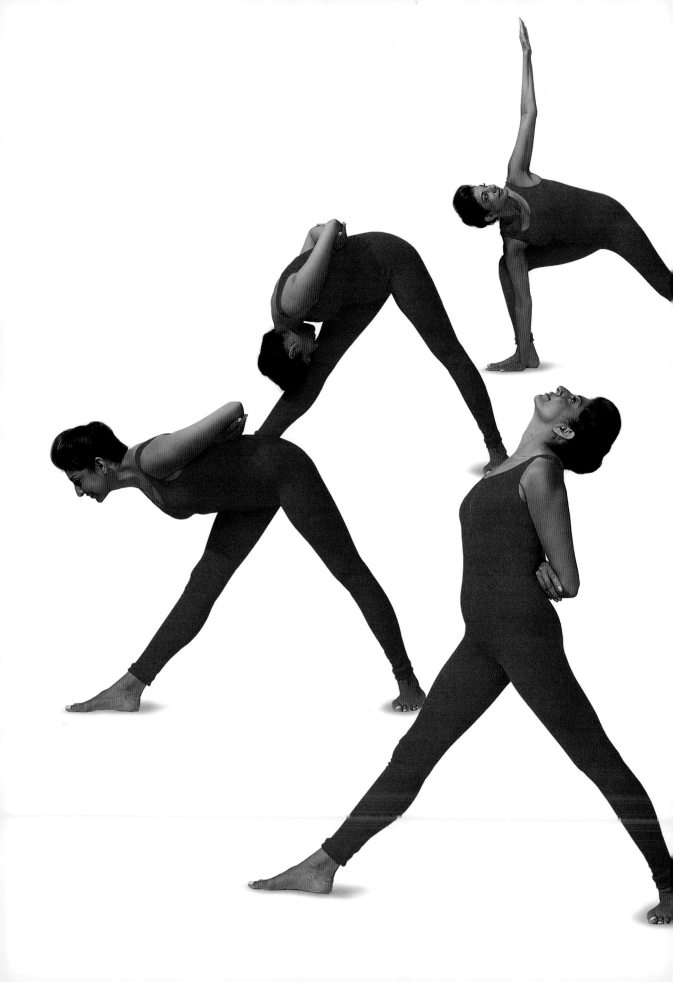

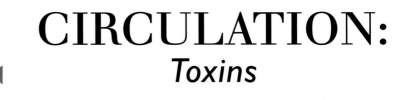

CIRCULATION:
Toxins

In yoga exercises, bending forward, sideways and backward allows every nerve, tissue and vein in the body to be replenished with fresh blood and oxygen. This purifies the system, releasing any harmful toxins that have become trapped. When you do this dynamic exercise you might think that you are simply perspiring, but you are actually eliminating toxins from your body. Some people may feel ill while exercising because drinking alcohol, using drugs, stress and bad eating habits all contribute to toxin buildup. If toxins are not removed, the immune system can break down, leading to serious illnesses such as heart disease, ulcers and diabetes.

This exercise is a continuation of the one given on the previous page, so you begin it from position 5.

With your right knee still bent, inhale and take your hand down to the floor in front of your right foot. As you exhale, twist your body around so your shoulders are in line. ▶Inhale, take your left arm up in the air with your palm facing back and continue to twist, looking over your left shoulder. Exhale and breathe normally. Straighten your arm and look upward toward the palm. ▶Turn back toward your right leg, straighten your knee and clasp both elbows behind your back. Drop your forehead down to the knee. Breathe deeply and hold for 5 to 10 seconds. ▶Inhale, and bring your body up so that your back is flat. Exhale, and breathe deeply for 5 to 10 seconds. ▶Inhale, and bring your body up, then drop your head back to release your neck. Exhale, breathe normally and hold for 5 seconds. Repeat on the other side.

CIRCULATION:
Joints

This simple swinging of the arms and body helps to increase circulation, particularly in your joints, hands and fingertips. If you suffer from stress-related rheumatism and arthritis, this exercise will ease the pain because the circular swing gradually loosens the joints. Yoga with its gentle approach will help shift the stiffness while relaxing the muscle groups through correct breathing. If your hip, knee or elbow joints are acutely inflamed, never try to force any movement. Just gently ease into the swing, breathing deeply to relax your mind and mobilize your entire body. Keep your feet still as you move the body around from one side to another.

Stand upright with your legs 1m (3ft) apart, your toes pointing forward and your arms at the side. Turn your body to the right and look over your right shoulder with your arm in line with the shoulder. ▶Inhale and bring your right arm down. ▶Exhale and begin to swing your arm across the front of your body in a circular motion and back up until it is in a diagonal line to your head, stretching to the left as you do so. While swinging, relax your knees and release your hips so that you have a wider swing. ▶Inhale, then as you exhale keep stretching to the left, while twisting your spine. Breathe normally and hold for 10 seconds. Repeat the whole exercise on the other side. Practice the swing on both sides a few times until you feel that all your joints have been loosened.

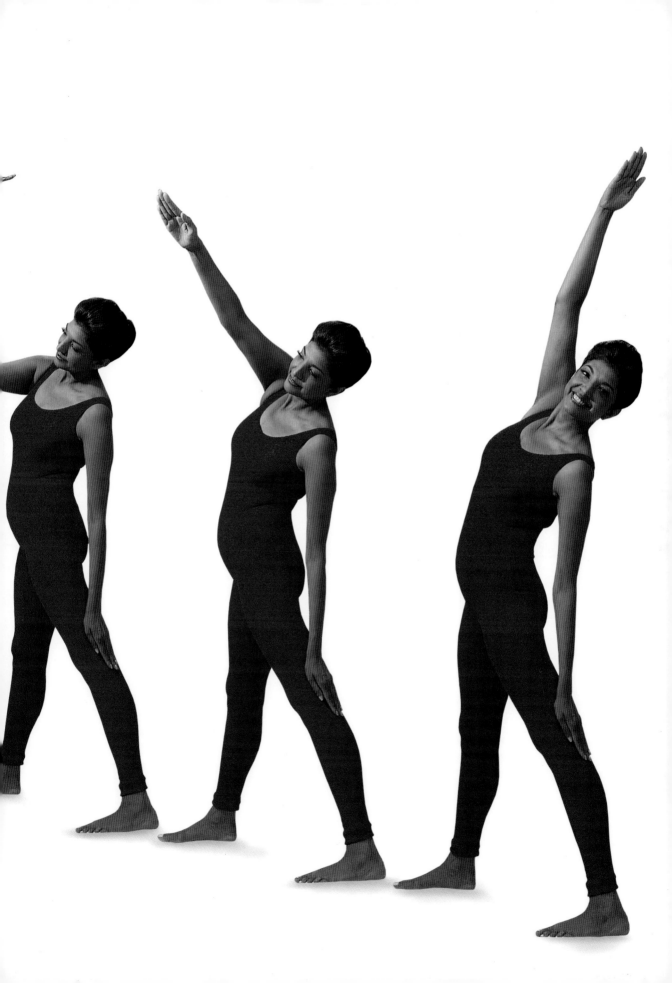

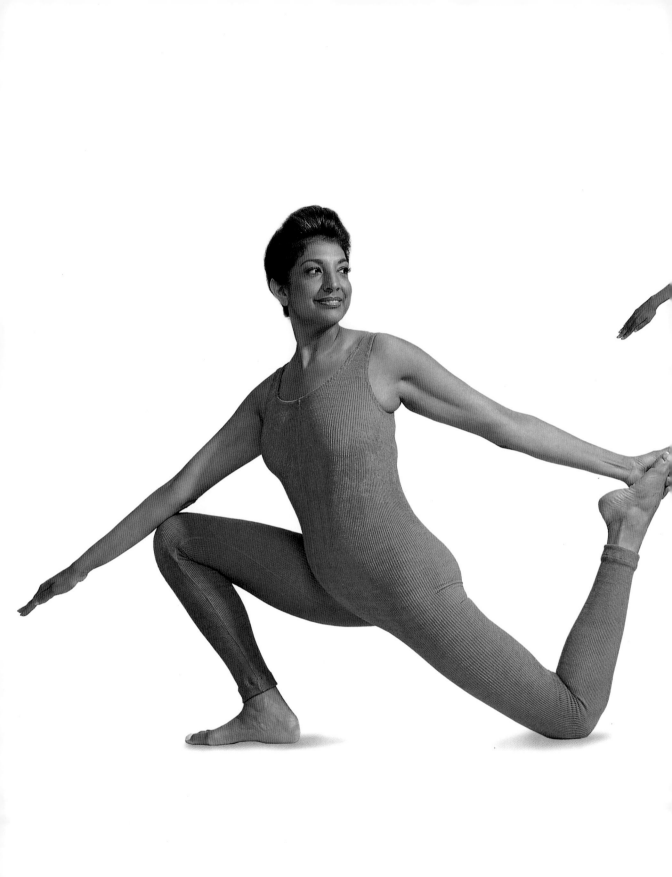

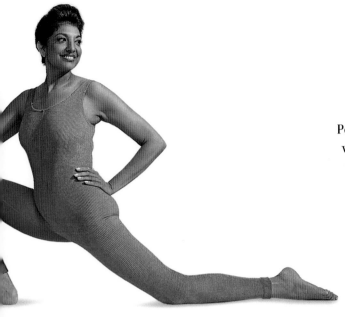

BACK:
Muscles

People who suffer from back pain are often worried that by exercising they will damage their backs even further. On the contrary, it is vital to strengthen back muscles in order to prevent strain and alleviate pain. Yoga provides a natural solution because of its emphasis on posture and correct alignment of the spine. While exercising you constantly build these muscles while noticing at all times the natural position of the spine. You are aware that in order to stand or sit in perfect posture the muscles of the lower back must support the rest of the spine. Sciatica and slipped discs are a result of weakness in the back, and a strong, healthy back is necessary for total body health.

This exercise tones and strengthens the back while helping to increase flexibility. It also shapes the waist, hips and legs.

Start by standing tall with both feet together. Inhale, and drop your head down to your knees. Exhale and bend both knees. Inhale, simultaneously straightening your left leg directly behind you while lunging forward with the right. Point your left foot and keep your hips and torso facing to the front. Inhale, slowly twist your upper body to the left and look over your left shoulder. ▶Now lift your left leg up and take hold of your toes. Exhale and balance for 5 seconds. Make sure that you are not balancing on your kneecap but on top of the knee to avoid any damage or strain. To release, turn to the front, place your fingertips on the floor and return to the start position. Repeat the exercise on the other side.

BACK:
Spasms

When people are stressed their muscles, ligaments and nerves are affected. The result is back spasms or muscular contractions which deplete energy and lead to general aches and pains. These twists relieve spasmodic tension while strengthening the muscles. Breathe deeply so your muscles relax and the spasms will cease. Be aware of your body's reactions; always listen to your body to remain healthy.

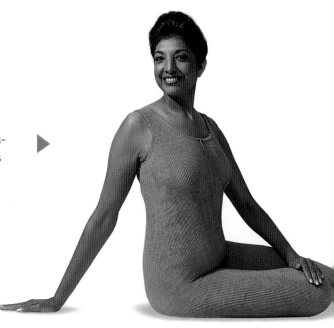

For the first twist, sit on your right hip with both legs bent to the left. Place your left hand on your right knee and take your right arm behind you. Inhale, twist to the right and look over your right shoulder. Exhale and breathe normally for 10 to 15 seconds. Repeat on the other side.

If you feel a sharp pain, stop twisting. A dull pain is fine provided it does not worsen.

For the second twist, sit up tall with both legs out in front of you, breathing normally. Bring your right foot in to the inner knee of your left leg. Lean forward, stretching from your tailbone. Flex your left thumb, bend your elbow and, clasping your big toe with your first two fingers, twist to the right. Take your right hand to your lower back, palm facing upward, and look over your right shoulder to stretch further. Breathe normally; hold for 10 to 20 seconds. Repeat on the other side.

For the third twist, bend your left leg under you, your knee in line with your left hip. Take your right leg in front of your left knee so your hips are square. Inhale, taking your left arm under the knee to increase the stretch. Use your hand behind you, palm down, for support. Exhale, look over your right shoulder and twist. Repeat on the other side.

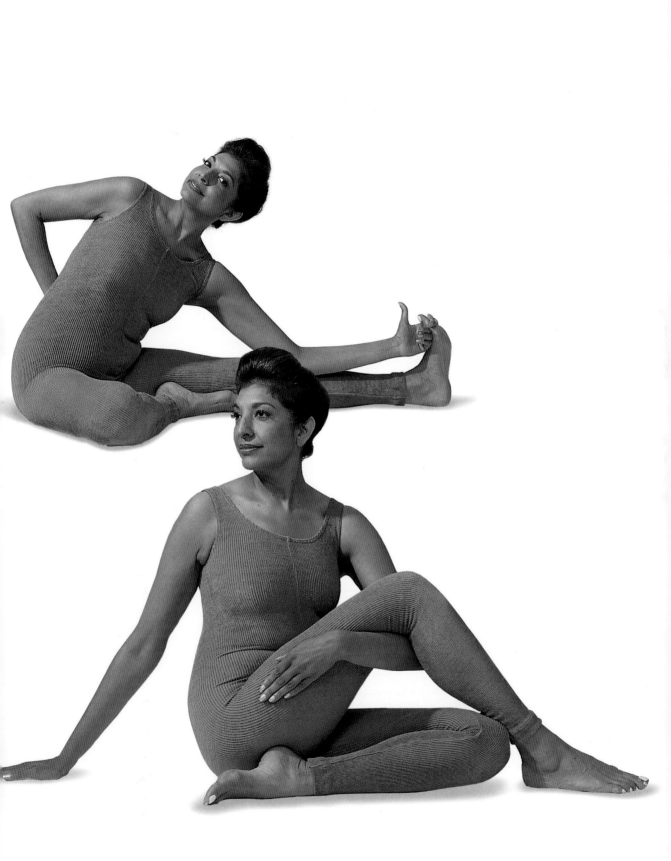

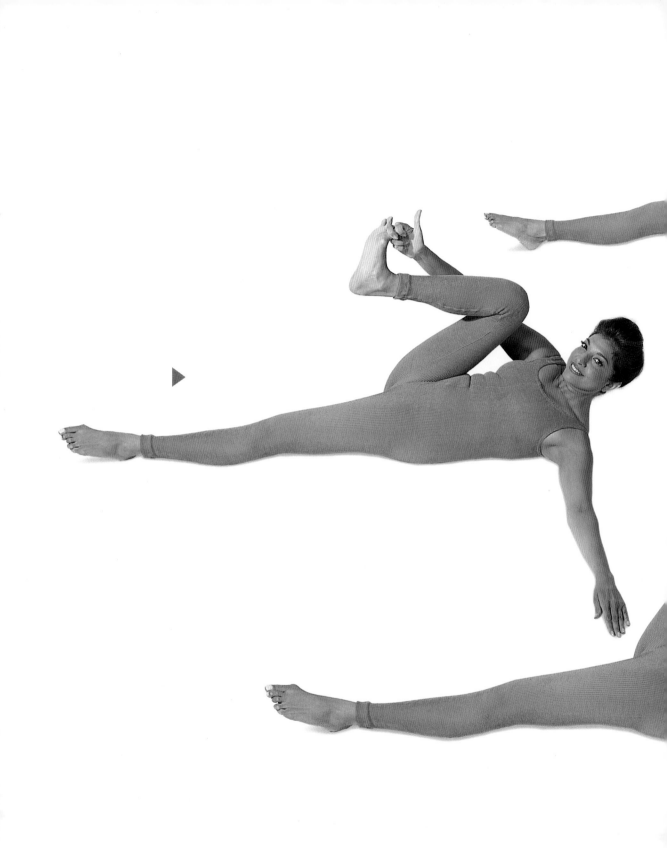

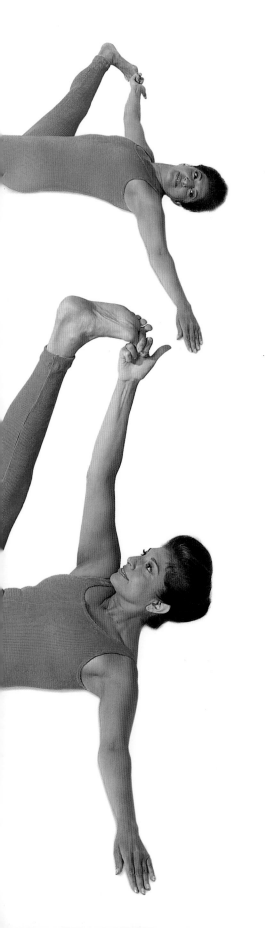

BACK:
Tension

Twisting laterally alleviates back pain while strengthening the lower back. If you feel any discomfort you can modify these positions by bending both knees throughout. Once you have a back ailment any tension will aggravate it, so try to keep mentally relaxed at all times. All stress manifests itself in your body and backs are particularly prone to chronic conditions. Yoga in its holistic approach is one of the best ways to cope with back ailments – relaxing and calming the mind and body eliminates emotions such as fear and anger which become trapped as tension in the muscle groups.

Start the exercise by lying flat on your back with your arms by your side. Take your arms out to the sides and put your palms face down on the floor, in line with your shoulders. Keeping your shoulders down, inhale and bend your right knee into your chest. Raise your head and, flexing your right thumb, clasp your big toe with your first two fingers. Make sure you keep your hips flat on the floor. ▶ Exhale and straighten the leg, still clasping your toe if you are able to. Hold for 5 seconds. Lower your head to the floor. ▶ Inhale again, and as you exhale take your leg to the right until it touches the floor at right angles to your body, still keeping your hips flat on the floor. Repeat the exercise on the other side.

ABDOMEN:
Stomach

Nervous tension in the stomach produces acidity, which can lead to gastric disorders such as flatulence, heartburn and irritable bowel syndrome. Acid or toxins begin to eat up the stomach lining, creating an imbalance which can result in these common ailments. Doctors now agree that there is a direct link between the emotional balance of a person and their susceptibility to certain illnesses. People suffering from stomach aches are often emotionally upset. The stomach can seize up with muscle cramps and most people take medication to relieve their pain. Yoga relaxes the stomach cramps immediately because it teaches you to breathe through the pain in order to release it.

Lie flat on the floor. Inhale and bring both knees into your chest, lifting your head off the floor. Exhale and breathe normally for 10 seconds. ▶Hold onto your right knee and place your left foot on the floor in front of your left hip. Inhale and bring your right knee closer in to your chest, pulling with your right hand on your knee and your left hand on your ankle. Exhale and hold for 5 seconds, breathing normally. ▶Take both hands around the back of your right knee, inhale deeply and exhale, straightening the right leg. Breathe normally and hold for 10 seconds. ▶Place your hands on your ankles, inhale and stretch your leg down toward your head. Exhale and bring your head up toward your leg. Breathe deeply and hold for 10 seconds, stretching until your forehead touches your knee. Release the leg down and repeat on other side.

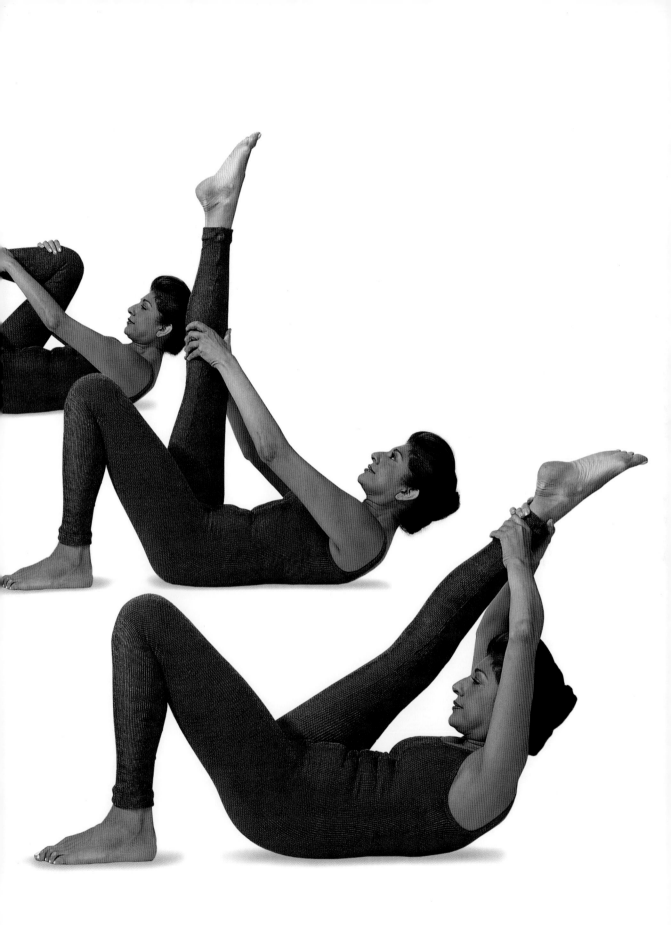

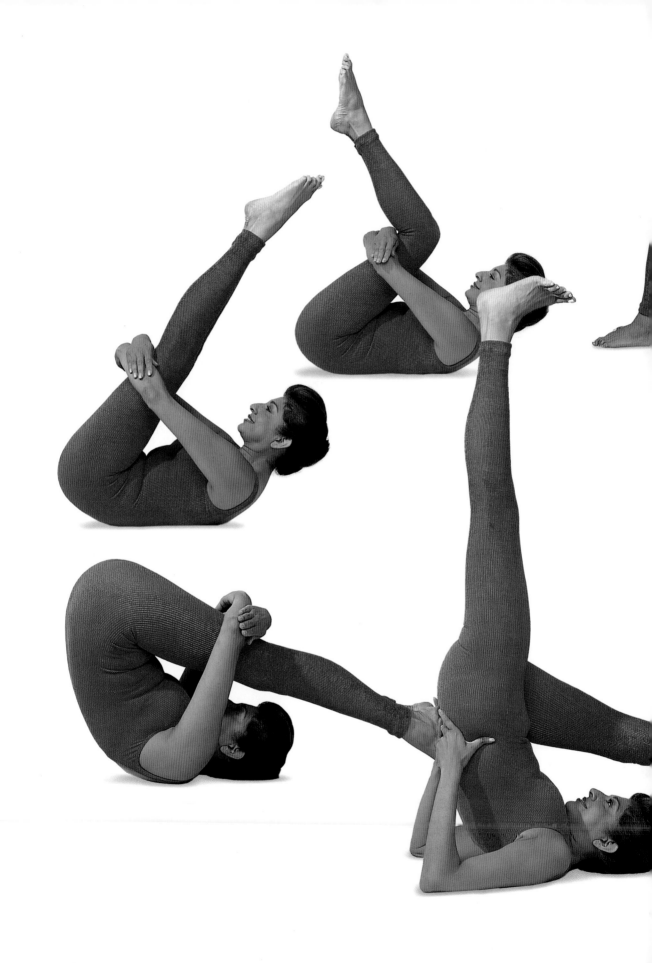

ABDOMEN:
Hormones

It is important to maintain a good hormonal balance during your life. At different phases of life, such as puberty, pregnancy or the menopause, hormone levels shift, causing emotional reactions and mood swings. Pre-menstrual syndrome is, in fact, more common today due to modern stress levels. Hormone replacements help, but can have side effects, whereas yoga naturally relieves the imbalance and stabilizes the hormonal levels. According to yogic texts when the head is locked into the chest it stimulates the thyroid gland, balancing your metabolism. If you are more than three months pregnant, do not take your legs over your head as this alters the position of the uterus.

Lie flat on the floor. Bring your knees up but keep your feet on the floor with your arms at your sides. ▶Inhale, bringing both knees into your chest, clasping your elbows under your knees. Exhale, lifting your head slightly off the floor. Breathe deeply; hold for 5 seconds. ▶ Breathe normally and straighten both legs, lifting your head up further. ▶ Take your hands to your waist for support and gently roll back, taking your legs over your head. Keep breathing deeply. Hold for 10 to 15 seconds. ▶Inhale, tuck your toes under and lift your left leg up straight. Exhale, then breathe normally; hold for 10 seconds. Inhale, exhale and lower your left leg down. Inhale, and raise your right leg. Exhale, and breathe normally for 10 seconds. Release both knees into your chest and roll back down to the start position.

RESPIRATION:
Stress

Ailments such as asthma and bronchitis are commonplace when stress factors affect the respiratory tract. Slowing your breathing down to an even pace while increasing the depth acts as a natural tranquillizer to the nervous system. Increasing your lung capacity also helps to relieve fatigue and hypertension that stems from breathing disorders. When people are fearful or panicky their heart races, their breathing becomes shallow and noisy, and they may pant. This exercise can help you to release tension and teaches you how to regulate your breathing pattern to reduce stress at a deeper level. You will then experience a sense of harmony and inner calm. Every time you repeat the exercise, breathe more deeply until you feel your lungs are filled to the brim.

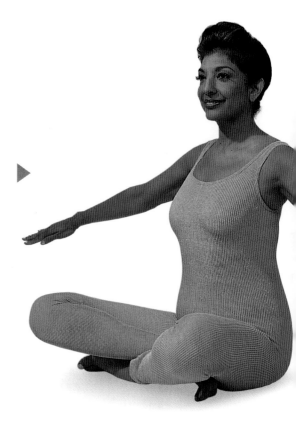

Sit comfortably in a cross-legged position on the floor, or upright in a chair with both feet flat on the floor. It is important that your spine stays straight and your head is in line with your neck and back. Concentrate on your navel and inhale deeply, taking your arms up slowly around your body. Feel the breath moving to fill your lungs. ▸Continuing to inhale, lift your arms up as you look upward. ▸Clasp your fingertips together and continue to stretch upward. Exhale and drop your head back, releasing your hands in a burst of energy. Repeat this exercise 5 to 10 times.

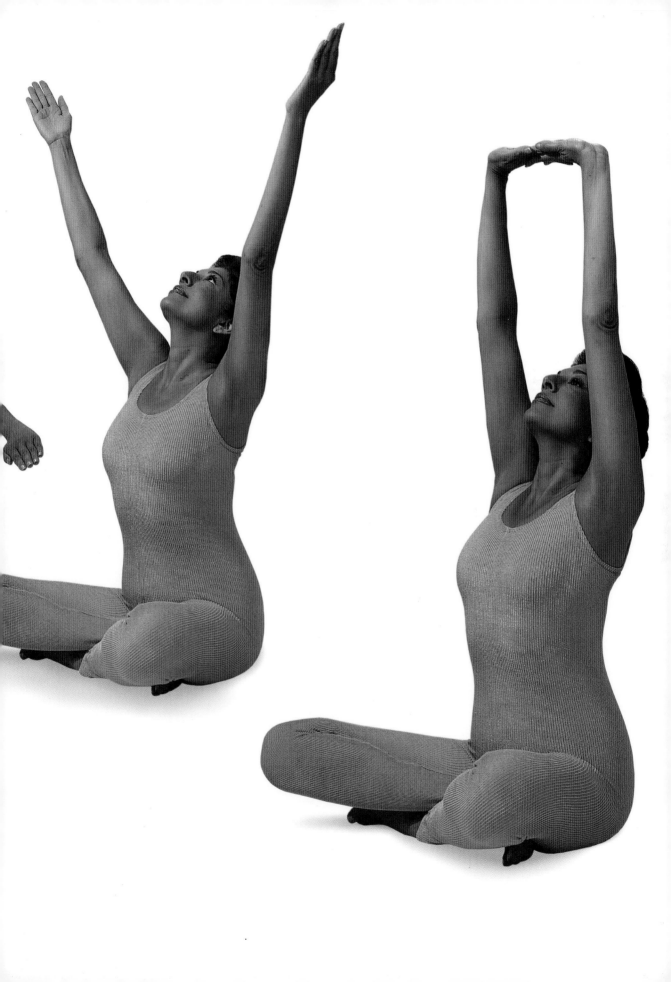

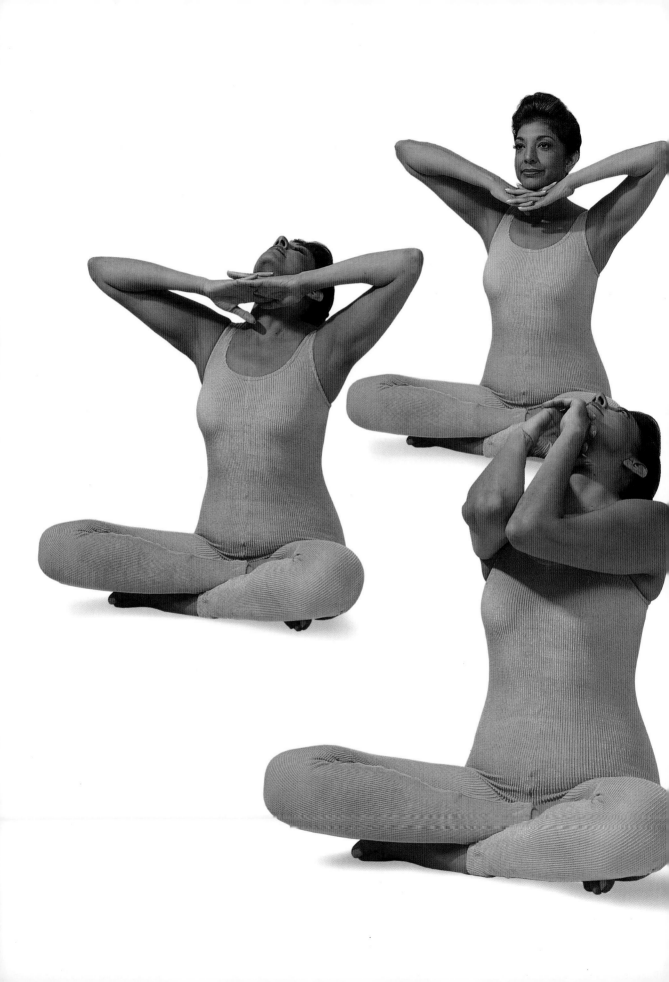

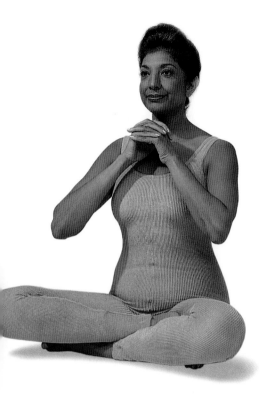

RESPIRATION:
Asthma

Bronchial asthma is a serious condition in which people suddenly experience difficulty in breathing. Their respiratory tract becomes blocked and they have great difficulty in exhaling. Panic sets in, along with a tight chest, coughing attacks and an audible wheezing. This breathing exercise is very helpful in preventing and reducing the severity of these attacks. Asthma can be triggered by allergies, smoking and pollution and is often linked to stress. Yoga breathing helps to calm the nervous system, reduce the emotional imbalances and restore body harmony.

Sit upright in a chair or on the floor in a comfortable cross-legged position. Clasp your fingertips together and place them under your chin. Make sure to keep your chin level and in a natural position to your neck. ▶Inhale deeply and raise your elbows as high as possible. ▶Holding your breath, drop your head back and take your elbows up level with your chin. ▶Leave your head back, exhale strongly and bring your elbows together. Inhale, return to position 2 and repeat the breathing pattern 10 to 20 times. If you are sitting on the floor, keep your knees down on the floor to increase your lung capacity.

RESPIRATION:
Panic

The ability to relax and control your breathing pattern helps to reduce fear during a panic attack. The bronchial tubes allow fresh oxygen into the lungs while dispelling carbon dioxide. When an attack is imminent, the muscles in the walls of the tubes constrict the breath flow. When you are particularly active you can hear the change in your breath as you need more air to sustain your activity. On the other hand, when you are resting or sleeping, little air is required. If you feel an attack coming on, take your mind off it and calm your nervous system by breathing from the diaphragm. The muscles of the bronchial tubes will relax as you allow more breath to enter your lungs and your mental state will improve as you realize that you are in control of every reaction to the attack.

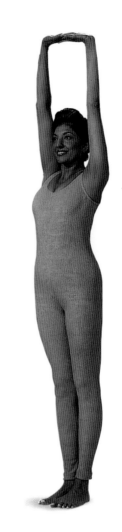

Stand tall in perfect posture. Stretch your arms high above your head, clasping your hands together. Keep your elbows straight and close to your ears. Force your shoulder blades down. Hold for 5 seconds, breathing normally. ▶Inhale, and rise up on your toes. Breathe deeply; hold for 5 seconds, concentrating on balancing. ▶Lift your heels higher, as you bend your knees. ▶Drop your heels down and stretch your hips backward as if reaching for a chair. The depth of your breathing will increase automatically. Keep your spine straight and your arms in line with your ears. Breathe deeply for 20 seconds. Repeat.

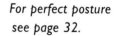

For perfect posture see page 32.

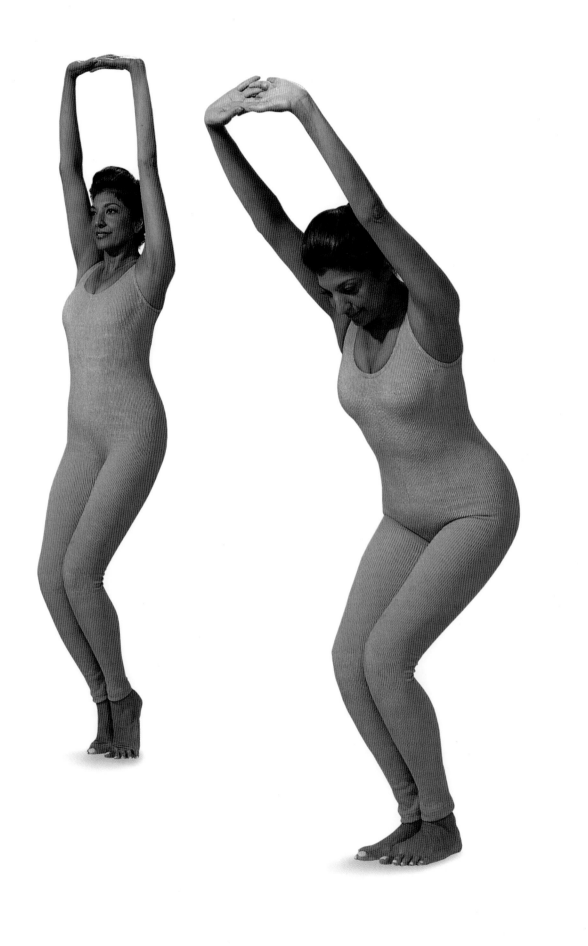

Index to exercises and ailments

ACKNOWLEDGEMENTS

Publishing Director:
Laura Bamford

Art Director:
Keith Martin

Senior Designer:
Ben Barrett

Designer:
Paul Webb

Commissioning Editor:
Jane McIntosh

Editors:
Mary Lambert   Diana Vowles

Production Controller:
Melanie Frantz

Photography:
John Adriaan

Hair and Make-up:
Leslie Sayles

Bodysuits kindly supplied by 'Sportique Fitness' UK.

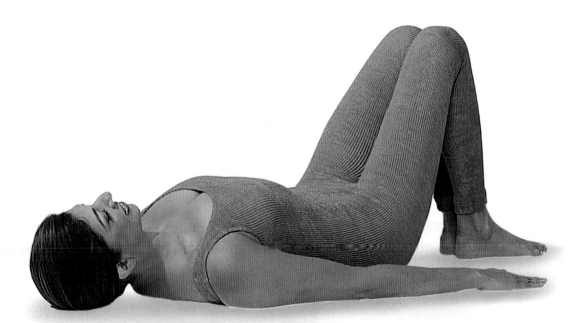